CONTENTS

From simple to science: why low carbohydrate diets work and how to practically apply them

INTELLIGENT

20 40.078	37 85.468
Ca	Rb

BETTER HEALTH FROM TWO MUSCULOSKELETAL EXPERTS

JOHN RIEHL, MD AND
JEFFREY LUTTON, MD

Year of the Book
135 Glen Avenue
Glen Rock, PA 17327

Print ISBN: 978-1-64649-143-8 (color)
Print ISBN: 978-1-64649-168-1 (b&w)
Ebook ISBN: 978-1-64649-144-5

This book is not intended as a substitute for the medical advice of your physician. The reader should regularly consult a physician in matters relating to his/her health and particularly with respect to any symptoms that may require diagnosis or medical attention.

INTRODUCTION

Low-carbohydrate diets have become increasingly popular over the past several years. Their popularity is largely a result of the fact that they work. While several variations of low-carbohydrate diets exist, few (if any) have been described by orthopaedic surgeons who see the end result of poor nutrition and an inactive lifestyle. From decreased mobility, to joint destruction, to loss of quality of life these effects are all too common in America today. We think our perspective is a valuable addition to the already existing body of knowledge to help people live the most active and fulfilling life possible.

For a lot of people, dieting is about much more than looking better; dieting can mean the difference between good health and chronic disease taking over their lives. Often times, specific diet plans are necessary to control chronic disease states and should be administered under the guidance of a trained professional. These diets may consist of different proportions of macronutrients based on the ability to metabolize certain molecules, or based on protein, vitamin, or other deficiencies that are a result of some underlying pathology.

For others, dieting really is more about feeling and looking better. It will also have the positive side effect of helping to prevent many common disease states from ever beginning. For healthy individuals, there are several diet options that can help to achieve weight loss/muscle building goals. Some of these options have been time tested and used successfully to accomplish these goals. The unfortunate truth that countless people experience, however, is that many diets work for a few weeks, or even a few months, but become difficult to provide a lasting benefit. This problem can often result from one of two issues: 1) failure to stick to an eating plan, or 2) the body's ability to adapt to a diet.

While the latest fad diet might help you lose weight initially, diets like these can be hard to stick with long term. When boredom with the new diet kicks in, or cravings for those foods you used to enjoy become too great and the luster from the fad diet has worn off, the urge to cheat can overpower even very strong-willed people. On the other hand, when first starting out with a new diet, strictly sticking to it can be interesting and fun. If you can capture that feeling with a safe and effective diet and keep it going, you can be successful in achieving your goals.

Additionally, the human body's ability to adapt is remarkable. The body can adapt to temperature changes, bones adapt to fractures by healing thicker and stronger with fracture callus, and muscles adapt to lifting heavy weights by getting bigger. The body adapts itself when faced with infection, and it can even adapt to changes in diet. Because of this ability to adapt, people can find themselves hitting plateaus with diets that previously provided significant gains.

Periodically changing diets, supplements, and exercise programs can therefore help avoid these two problems. In this book we will focus on low carbohydrate diets and explain some of the science behind why these diets work and their benefits, however we acknowledge the advantages to other types of diets and even the potential benefits to using some of them intermittently in order to keep yourself interested in eating healthy and preventing your body from adapting to any one specific diet.

1 | GETTING HEALTHY

Diets often fall short of helping people to reach their goals. But failure does not usually come from a poor diet plan (as many types of diets can be successful if strictly adhered to), rather it comes from incomplete dedication to getting healthy. In fact, many people fail to define for themselves from the outset what it means to "get healthy." It may mean something different for you than what it means for your friend, or co-worker, or spouse. Getting healthy might mean losing weight for some, while for others it means gaining weight. For most, however, getting healthier ultimately will result in losing fat while gaining lean muscle. Prior to beginning any diet plan it is important to clearly define your goals. Write them down and be specific. Attach dates to those goals as well as a plan of action. Doing this will help to increase your chances of success.

There are certain disease states as well that can be overcome with proper diet and exercise. For people with these diseases, such as diabetes and heart disease, getting healthy might be life-saving. Not only can a healthier lifestyle improve some disease states, but it can also certainly help prevent disease. Many people right now are on the borderline for diagnoses of chronic diseases such as diabetes and high blood pressure. They are trying to "diet" as an attempt to control these diseases and avoid taking medications that have significant side effects. Unfortunately, many people in this situation will ultimately see their disease progress, their "diet control" attempt fail, and they are left with no other option than to begin expensive and life-altering medication regimens. Often, this diet control failure results from two main reasons. First, patients are often told to "eat healthy" without being given the proper direction on exactly how to do that. Traditional low-fat and low-calorie diets fall short in a multitude of ways for people trying to avoid disease progression. As you will see in this book, carbohydrates and carbohydrate metabolism can cause several effects on a cellular level (i.e. inside the body's cells) that can allow disease progression despite the best of efforts. Second, many "traditional diets" leave people feeling hungry, which most people will only tolerate for so long. As a human being you have natural instincts. One of those instincts is to eat when you're hungry. You may be able to overcome this instinct consistently for a few weeks, or even a few months. Long term though, who wants to feel hungry all the time? Carbohydrates (specifically, simple carbohydrates) increase the sensation of hunger. As time goes on you are susceptible to overeat and lose what health gains you have made on high carbohydrate diets.

BIOCHEMICAL EFFECTS OF CARBOHYDRATES

If scientific terms make you cringe or make your eyes gloss over, it is okay to skip this section. It has been placed here for those who are interested in a brief overview of the biochemical effect carbohydrates (and the lack thereof) have on your body. It is not essential to know this information in order to follow a ketogenic diet or a diet consisting of intelligent carbohydrate sources, but it does provide some of the basic science knowledge as to why this all works in your body.

Carbohydrates (shortened to carbs, and throughout this book also referred to as sugars) are molecules that are made up of carbon, hydrogen, and oxygen. Glucose is what is known as a simple carbohydrate and is one of the main sources of fuel used by your body. Glucose is present in a variety of foods and can be ingested directly or it will be ultimately what many carbohydrates are turned into prior to being absorbed in your intestinal tract. Glucose is used by muscle, liver, and brain cells to power their cellular functions. Let's take a brief look at what happens to a carbohydrate from the moment it is eaten until it is used as energy by a muscle cell or stored for later use.

When you take a bite of a slice of pizza, the mechanical act of chewing begins to break up the bite into pieces small enough to swallow. At the same time, saliva begins to mix with the food pieces and begins the digestive process. Saliva contains proteins called enzymes that help with this process.

When you swallow, the food travels down the esophagus (the tube connecting your mouth to your stomach) and muscle contractions in the walls of the esophagus help to bring food down to the stomach.

Once in the stomach, food particles are mixed with additional enzymes and acid that further break down the molecules in the food. Food is held in the stomach and mixes in this chemical stew until it is broken down enough to be released into the intestine.

The intestine is divided into two main segments: the small intestine, and the large intestine. The stomach is connected to the small intestine which is roughly 20 feet long and 1 inch in diameter, while the large intestine adds another 5 feet to this system at 3 inches in diameter. The small intestine is further divided into three parts termed the duodenum, jejunum, and ileum. As food leaves the stomach and enters the small intestine, new enzymes are added to the mix by the pancreas and the liver. All the while muscular contractions in the walls of the intestine continue to mix and move food along. In the first portion of the small intestine (duodenum), many of the large and medium sized molecules will be broken down to component molecules that become dissolved into the surrounding liquid and can be absorbed through the intestinal wall and into the bloodstream. Food particles that do not get absorbed while in the small intestine will continue to pass through into the large intestine, and in large part will ultimately be excreted.

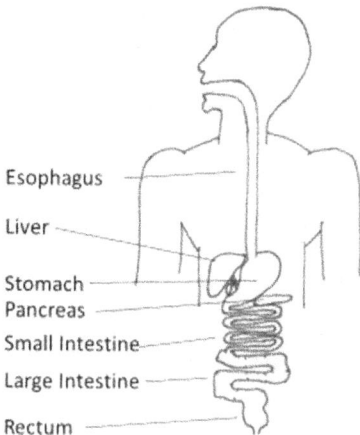

Esophagus

Liver

Stomach
Pancreas

Small Intestine

Large Intestine

Rectum

- Digestion begins with food being chewed and combined with enzymes in saliva
- Food is brought down the esophagus through the coordinated action of smooth muscles (peristalsis)
- Further mixing of food and addition of more digestive enzymes occurs in the stomach (acidic environment)
- Carbohydrate chains are suspended in solution as they leave the stomach
- Smaller food particles enter into the small intestine. Enzymes from the liver and pancreas are released. Long carbohydrate chains are broken down into 2-sugar chains and ultimately into single sugars (monosaccharides). These single sugars are then absorbed through the wall of the small intestine
- Once in the bloodstream, the monosaccharide glucose can be taken up by cells for use as energy and will stimulate the pancreas to release insulin

Figure 1.1—Glucose Digestion

Throughout this process, the enzymes involved are breaking up the carbohydrates in that slice of pizza from one large chain of sugar molecules strung together into the individual smaller component parts of that chain. By the time that pizza has bathed in the acids of the stomach and is making its way into the duodenum, many of the carbohydrate chains are suspended in liquid form and are acted upon by an enzyme from the pancreas called pancreatic amylase, which breaks the large chain of sugars into chains of just two sugars. Other enzymes within the small intestine then further breakdown the two sugar chains into single sugars (called monosaccharides) that are then absorbed through the wall of the small intestine and enter into the bloodstream. Among these single sugar molecules is glucose.

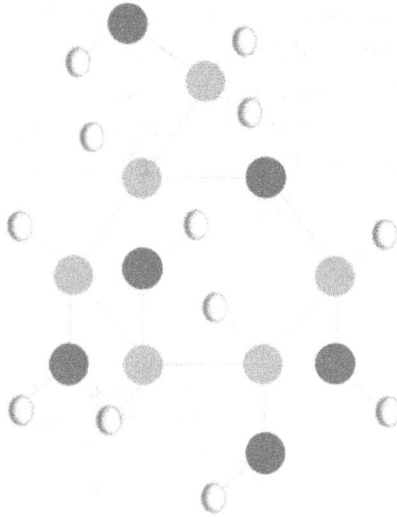

Figure 1.2—Glucose

Once in the bloodstream, glucose molecules can be transported to cells for use as energy or can be taken up by the liver and muscle and stored for later use.

As blood glucose levels (blood sugar levels) rise, this stimulates the pancreas to release insulin. The more rapid and the greater the amount of glucose that is absorbed into the bloodstream, the greater the insulin response will be. Once insulin is released into the bloodstream, it signals cells to allow glucose to enter into them.

Effects of Insulin

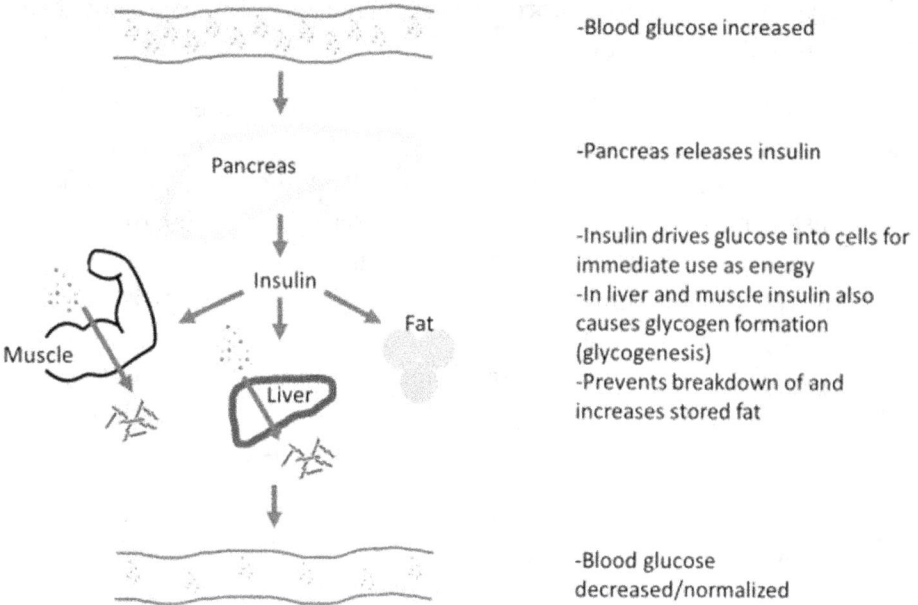

-Blood glucose increased

-Pancreas releases insulin

-Insulin drives glucose into cells for immediate use as energy
-In liver and muscle insulin also causes glycogen formation (glycogenesis)
-Prevents breakdown of and increases stored fat

-Blood glucose decreased/normalized

Figure 1.3—Glucose Storage and Muscle Utilization: Effects of Insulin

In addition to providing an immediate glucose supply to cells, the insulin sends signals to convert the excess glucose into storage for later use.

In liver and muscle cells, this excess glucose is stored in a form of multiple glucose molecules linked together called glycogen.

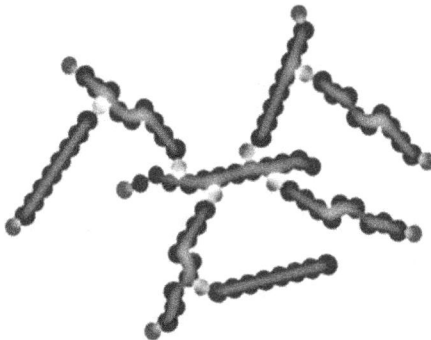

Figure 1.4—Glycogen

Glycogen is a form of energy storage that can be quickly converted back into glucose when blood sugar levels are low, and energy is needed. However, when glycogen stores are in full supply, the excess glucose circulating in the blood will be turned into adipose tissue (fat).

While there is a limit to how much glycogen can be stored in the body, fat can be stored in extremely large quantities. Fatty acids can be used as an energy source for cells at times as well. When blood sugar levels are raised, however, the body prevents breakdown of fat for use as energy because it is not needed with circulating glucose present to be used as the energy source for cells. Therefore, when energy is needed in the body, glucose is the first choice, followed by glycogen, and finally fat. This, of course, is an oversimplification of the complex processes that are occurring in your body every day, but enough of an explanation to give you a general picture of what is going on.

When insulin is circulating in the system, therefore, fat will not be broken down and used as an energy source. Before you blame insulin for your excess fat stores, however, we need to pause and observe that insulin is not the enemy, but rather is a necessity when blood sugar levels are high.

Without insulin, circulating glucose would remain elevated for long periods and would be accompanied by severe consequences which are beyond the scope of this book, but ultimately can lead to problems such as peripheral vascular disease, kidney disease, stroke, heart attack, nerve pain, ulcers, infections, loss of limb, etc. Emerging research shows there is often evidence of disordered glucose metabolism long before diabetes results. Fasting insulin levels may be a more sensitive way to detect these metabolic abnormalities than fasting glucose levels. As long as glucose is available under normal conditions it will be used as the source of energy before fat stores will get used. Therefore, avoiding spikes in blood glucose is a key component to getting rid of that excess fat.

As a result of the science behind glucose metabolism that has just been described, eating plans that attempt to keep spikes in blood glucose from occurring can be completely derailed by foods that cause brief, large increases in blood sugar during the day. In other words, sneaking some potato chips in the afternoon will prevent weight loss on a low carb diet because it will prevent your body from using up fat stores. By providing your body with glucose and causing the resultant insulin spikes, fat stores stay put. While those potato chips might not seem like a significant cheat, they will halt fat loss by causing glucose absorption and a spike in blood sugar.

Next, let's look at what happens when glucose is in short supply (i.e., low blood sugar, or when you have swapped out that pizza for chicken).

Brain cells are heavily dependent upon glucose for energy. The human body must, therefore, have a mechanism to supply these cells with glucose in times where glucose is not being ingested (for example, when sleeping, fasting, on a low carb diet, etc.).

When blood sugar levels are low, glucagon (another hormone from the pancreas) is released. Glucagon has the opposite effect of insulin, in that it raises the amount of glucose circulating in the blood. Glucagon stimulates the breakdown and release of stored glucose (called glycogen) and stimulates a process whereby glucose can be made from other molecules (called gluconeogenesis).

Because gluconeogenesis uses protein (in addition to other non-carbohydrate molecules) to make glucose, increased protein ingestion will help to prevent depletion of protein (and muscle) in the body. In this state of low carbohydrate ingestion, glucose is therefore still provided for the cells that need it.

Glucose will preferentially be taken up by brain cells because insulin is not required for glucose to travel into brain cells, as is required for some other cell types. Additionally, glucagon signals the breakdown of fatty acids to be used for energy, which ultimately can have a desirable effect on the size pants you buy.

Effects of Glucagon

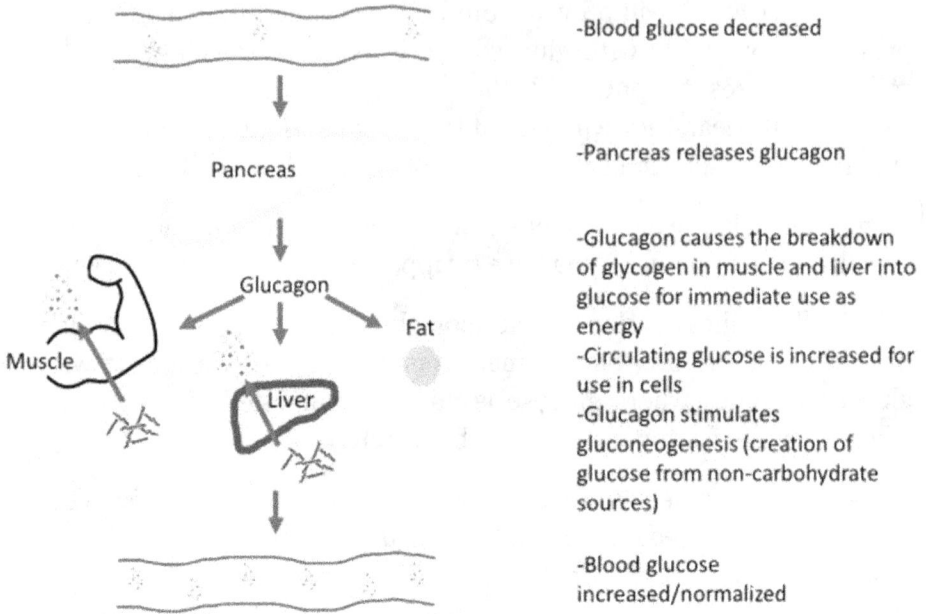

-Blood glucose decreased

Pancreas

-Pancreas releases glucagon

Glucagon

Muscle

Fat

Liver

-Glucagon causes the breakdown of glycogen in muscle and liver into glucose for immediate use as energy
-Circulating glucose is increased for use in cells
-Glucagon stimulates gluconeogenesis (creation of glucose from non-carbohydrate sources)

-Blood glucose increased/normalized

Figure 1.5—Glucose Storage and Muscle Utilization: Effects of Glucagon

The last related process to carbohydrate metabolism that is worth mentioning here is ketosis. Ketosis can be a dangerous condition when present in diabetic patients and can even become life-threatening (referred to as diabetic ketoacidosis). This condition is characterized by acid buildup and typically occurs in Type I diabetics with severely elevated blood sugar levels. Ketosis can also be a beneficial byproduct of a low carbohydrate diet, whereby ketone bodies are formed (sometimes referred to as nutritional ketosis). Ketone bodies are made from fatty acids and are formed in the liver when glycogen stores are depleted. Ketone bodies can then be taken up by cells and used as fuel to produce energy to power cellular functions. Ketogenic diets have been used for medical purposes dating back to the ancient Greeks and became popular as a treatment for epilepsy as far back as the 1920s. Several recent studies have shown positive effects of ketogenic diets including weight loss, decreasing cardiovascular disease risk, improvement in hemoglobin A1C levels (marker of diabetes disease progression), and lowered blood pressure.[1-4]

EFFECT OF INSULIN RESISTANCE ON MUSCLE
– INTERMUSCULAR ADIPOSE TISSUE (IMAT)

As surgeons, we strive for perfect patient outcomes with every surgery we perform. Despite our best efforts, some people seem to heal and recover much faster than others. We go through the same steps, apply the same surgical techniques, prescribe the same post-operative rehab, but we do not see consistent results between all patients. It is our belief that disordered glucose metabolism has a negative effect on skeletal muscle, bones, and may be responsible (at least in part) for the varied response to surgery.

One of the principles of orthopedic surgery is to restore anatomy. Whether it is reconstructing a knee ligament or repairing a fractured shin bone, we strive to restore the extremities to a nondiseased state. When the structure of a bone is disturbed, a change in function usually follows. Structural changes within muscle can cause changes in function also. There is an associated decrease in strength with decreasing muscle mass, typically seen with advancing age. Intermuscular adipose tissue (IMAT) is a change in the quality and quantity of muscle that can be seen in various medical conditions including stroke and spinal cord injury. Insulin resistance and diabetes has more recently been implicated as a cause of IMAT.[5]

IMAT is the presence of fat in an unusual location. Most fat is found just below the skin in the subcutaneous tissue. IMAT is found beneath fascia (a covering of muscle tissue) and within skeletal muscle. High levels of IMAT are associated with insulin resistance and diabetes.[6] IMAT has been correlated with loss of strength, mobility, function, and subsequently decreased quality of life. In contrast to IMAT, a different method of fat storage is found in endurance runners called intramyocellular lipids (IMCL). Fat is stored in the muscle cells themselves and is not harmful to the structure or function of the muscle.

Skeletal muscle is the number one user of glucose. Not surprisingly, IMAT has been associated with disordered glucose metabolism (insulin resistance). We currently do not know if IMAT is a cause of these problems, or the result of impaired glucose metabolism. There may be a vicious cycle of impaired metabolism leading to impaired function, which leads to less muscle activity and impaired metabolism.

Ectopic fat (fat in places it doesn't belong, such as in the liver or around other abdominal organs) releases signaling molecules that cause inflammation. There is evidence this is also the case with IMAT.[7]

We mentioned earlier that decreased muscle mass is seen with advancing age. Surprisingly, the decrease in strength is more than would be expected from the loss of muscle alone.[8] There is therefore likely something else that should explain this additional loss of strength. The change in muscle structure seen with IMAT can help explain this discrepancy.

IMAT has been measured by CT scans as well as MRI. Interestingly, people of the same gender, age, BMI, and lean muscle mass but different amounts of IMAT have different strength. People who have less IMAT can produce more force per unit of muscle.[9] Clearly, the altered structure of muscle with IMAT decreases the quality of muscle.

Isolated muscle weakness from IMAT seems bad enough, but the result of this on all of your muscles working together is much worse. As orthopedic surgeons, our job is to reduce pain and improve function. IMAT greatly inhibits function by all objective measures. Some tests used to measure function are six-minute walking distance, gait speed, repeated chair stands, ascending stairs, and get up and go tests. Performance in all of these tests are worse with increasing IMAT.[10] IMAT can also be used to predict future disability, as those with higher IMAT have higher disability over a two-and-a-half-year period.

IMAT is also a predictor of osteoporosis and hip fractures. We have extensive experience treating fractures, and as we will discuss further, some bones are soft and brittle while others are healthy and supportive. It is interesting that, even when taking bone density into account, IMAT by itself is related to an increased risk of fracture.[11] Hip fractures are life-altering injuries and are best avoided. If the risk can be lessened by decreasing IMAT, some of the morbidity occurring every year around the world from hip fractures could be avoided.

What can be done about IMAT? Intentional weight loss decreases IMAT.[12] Equally active old and young people have the same degree of IMAT.[13] It is our opinion that by combining optimized glucose metabolism with regular strength training, the risk of IMAT and its associated decrease in function can be mitigated.

HOW DO I CHOOSE A DIET?

There are many types of diets out there, so how do you know which one to start? First, you need to look at diets that are actually going to produce the desired results when you follow them strictly. Some are designed for weight loss, some are designed to lower cholesterol, and some are designed with unrealistic expectations that can make them exceedingly difficult and expensive to stick with. Most people would be happy on a diet where they could eat their favorite foods all the time in whatever quantity they desire, however that is not conducive to fat loss and muscle building.

Your eating plan will have to restrict something from your diet. There are many diets that can produce desired results when followed appropriately, and we are not here to tell you that there's one eating plan that's best for everyone (although we will contend that for most people, a high protein and low carbohydrate diet will be beneficial compared to low fat and low-calorie diets). In fact, we will go one step further and say that there is not even necessarily one eating plan that's right for one person throughout their lifetime. The key is to choose a diet and exercise plan that works and one that you can follow to transform your health. If, throughout the course of that eating plan, you find that despite strictly following it you are not achieving your desired results, then you should change your approach.

You must honestly evaluate whether or not you are following your diet plan. A candy bar or a soda here or there can be the difference between a diet succeeding or failing, even if you're staying strict at mealtime. It is important to realize that this change in diet is part of a lifestyle change. You will fail at times. A minor slip up does not ruin a diet, but letting that turn into a two-week binge can undo months of progress. When your willpower fails, recognize it and get back on track.

It's important to make clear that we believe that this style of eating is not the only way to get healthy. For some people, it might not even be the best way. You can certainly lose weight on low-calorie diets and other portion control diet plans. The important thing is to find a healthy way of eating that works for you, and that you can use as part of a long-term strategy to a healthy life. For us (two guys who love to eat), we believe that an Intelligent Carb lifestyle allows you to eat good foods without having to feel hungry, while improving your health in a sustainable manner.

One common criticism of low carbohydrate diets is that once the diet is stopped and an individual returns to a "normal diet," weight tends to be regained. We would interpret this not as a criticism of low carb diets specifically, but rather an indictment of the standard high carb, highly processed American diet. A return to this type of diet from any successful eating program is likely to result in weight gain. Perhaps for most people it is best to think of an Intelligent Carb eating plan not as a "diet" but as a lifestyle change.

COMPLETE DEDICATION

Dieting success is not so different from success in sports, or school, or many other aspects of life. The foundation of success in personal health begins with planning and dedication to succeed. The first question to ask yourself is "why?" Why are you trying to get healthier? Is it to cure disease? Live a longer life? Be a better athlete? To look better in a bathing suit? Get specific with your answer to "why." Is your weight stopping you from playing with grandchildren? Is your health goal to avoid having to start giving yourself insulin shots? Do you want to gain 10 pounds of muscle so you can knock down anyone in your way on the football field? Whatever your reasons, find them and clearly articulate them from the beginning. Write them down. We recommend purchasing a composition notebook that you use to keep and track your reasons, your goals, your personal health statistics, and any other notes that you find useful on your journey to lifelong health. We recommend that you search for three "why's" that motivate you to get healthier. These "why's" will help define what getting healthy means to you. Have a clear definition that you put in writing.

Once you have done this, your next step is goal setting. Imagine what you want to achieve with good health. Your goals should be consistent with your "why," and the language describing the two may even overlap a little. Determine three long-term goals (big things that will take more than a couple months or even a year or more to achieve), and three short-term goals (things to achieve this week). Short-term goals should be made every week, along with an analysis of how well you achieved your goals from the previous week. Long-term goals should be re-evaluated from time to time and honest self-analysis of your progress toward those goals should be performed on a weekly basis.

Successfully getting healthy requires so much more than being told what to eat and when to exercise. It is truly a decision that comes from within you – a decision to change your life for the better. A decision that the sacrifice of not eating some of the foods you love to eat is worth it to ultimately feel better in your day to day life. And you will feel better as you shed fat, gain muscle, and improve your overall health. Even small amounts of weight loss can make a significant difference. For example, many people are not aware of this, but every 10 pounds of weight translates to somewhere around 30 pounds of force across your weight-bearing surface of your knee when climbing and descending stairs,[14] and may be even higher across your kneecap. Even if you don't see much of a difference in the mirror or in your waist size with the loss of 10 pounds, your joints will thank you at the end of the day for relieving them of their 30-pound burden with each step. It all starts with a strong desire within yourself to make a change, definitively deciding that you are going to go through with it, and cutting out all possibilities in your mind of failure.

In the beginning, it is important to get rid of, or keep out of sight, foods that might tempt you that you should not be eating. As time goes on, your cravings for these foods will diminish. You will notice how much better you feel without these foods, and your desire to eat them will decrease the longer you go without them. In much the same way that a person who quit smoking 30 years ago has very little to no desire for a cigarette today, you will begin in a few months to feel very little desire for high carbohydrate foods. Your early dedication will pay off and will make it easier for you to roll your short-term successes into long-term lifestyle changes.

The next two chapters will contain specific information on two eating styles that, when followed accurately, will help you to lose fat and gain muscle. Chapter 5 contains exercise programs that can be tailored to fit into any schedule. Recipes that fit into one or both of these diets can be found in Chapter 7.

2 | CARBS AND THE KETOGENIC DIET

OVERVIEW

The modern western diet has contributed substantially to a host of medical issues. In this diet, calories are drawn from primarily red meat, dairy, processed, and artificially sweetened foods. Fruit, vegetable, and legume consumption is less than it should be. This diet has been implicated in diabetes, cancer, cardiovascular disease, and neurodegenerative disease. The common pathway is poor regulation of glucose metabolism leading to protein glycosylation, increased body fat, and inflammation. In simple terms, this diet of refined carbohydrates and sugar is slowly killing us. In this chapter we will show how a low carbohydrate diet can improve glucose metabolism and lead to a healthier life.

WHY HIGH CARB CAN BE DETRIMENTAL

Evolutionarily, food was scarce. We ate what we could, and the digestive system evolved to maximize the extraction and storage of energy. As food production, storage, and distribution was mastered, humans (generally speaking) now have an overabundance of food. The excess carbohydrates present in most processed foods today have taken advantage of our body's efficient energy storage mechanisms to significantly contribute to our obesity problem.

Once entered into the body, nearly all carbohydrates that will be absorbed are eventually metabolized to glucose. This leads to the release of insulin from the Islet cells of the pancreas. Insulin is a complex hormone that influences our metabolism. Put simply, insulin signals cells to use glucose as the primary fuel source, and to store excess glucose as fat.

When a lot of glucose is consumed (as happens with drinking a large soda), a lot of insulin will be released. This will then lower the blood glucose by signaling cells in the muscle and liver to take glucose into the cell. So what's the problem? It's not really a problem when low to moderate amount of carbohydrates are consumed. The system begins to get overwhelmed, however, when higher amounts of carbohydrates are introduced.

High carbohydrate diets lead to higher levels of glucose and insulin in the bloodstream. High carbohydrate diets provide more glucose than is necessary. As mentioned earlier, insulin signals cells to take glucose into the cell to use as fuel. When the cell has all the glucose it can take, excess glucose is stored as glycogen in the liver and in muscle. When the cells in the liver and muscle are "full" of glycogen, the excess glucose is then stored as fat.

Fat storage isn't limited to what we can see on the outside of our bodies. Fat can be subcutaneous or visceral. Subcutaneous is the fat we see (and want to get rid of). Visceral fat is stored inside our abdomen around our organs. Visceral fat not only contributes to our large bellies, but is also extremely dangerous to our health. It is implicated in many chronic diseases including cardiovascular, neurodegenerative diseases, cancer, diabetes, and others. Fat does more than store calories. It also secretes hormones and pro-inflammatory signaling molecules called cytokines. Visceral fat can dump these hormones directly into the liver, contributing to insulin-resistance and "fatty-liver" formation.[15]

The pro-inflammatory cytokines released by visceral fat contribute to cardiovascular disease[16] and are a marker of general metabolic dysfunction. The hormonal changes brought about by visceral fat have been implicated in dementia and other neurodegenerative diseases.[17] There is even an association with visceral fat and depression in middle-aged women.

Fat will always be an available storage facility for extra energy, but in some metabolic conditions the signals to store glucose are overwhelmed and the receptors are downregulated (lowers the cell response to insulin). This causes a "backup" of glucose in the bloodstream. One way to better understand this is to examine what happens when insulin does not work.

DIABETES

Type 1 diabetes occurs when the body does not produce insulin. Glucose is absorbed from the gut into the bloodstream. Normally insulin would be released, and cells would respond by taking glucose in from the bloodstream. Because no insulin is produced, glucose builds up to dangerously high levels. This can cause damage to organs and lead to major medical complications such as peripheral vascular disease, retinal (eye) disease, heart disease, kidney disease, etc.

Type 2 diabetes is different. The primary problem is insulin resistance. Cells adapt to an abundance of glucose and glycogen. Essentially, the system is overwhelmed. The precise cause of this remains unknown, but the muscle and liver do not respond to insulin appropriately. The result is glucose backing up in the bloodstream.

Chronically elevated glucose levels lead to glycosylation of proteins (think about the sticky residue juice leaves on anything it touches). This is the reason for the observed increase in neuropathy (peripheral nerve problems), kidney problems, heart disease, and cancer in diabetics. One logical answer to this problem is to consume fewer carbohydrates.

Insulin also affects fat metabolism. When glycogen reserves are full, insulin triggers the liver to make fatty acids. These fatty acids are transported in the blood as lipoproteins (HDL, LDL, and others). The more the glucose/insulin pathway is turned on, the more lipids can enter the bloodstream. This has implications for development of atherosclerosis, or heart disease.

Perhaps most importantly from the standpoint of changing body composition and eliminating body fat, insulin prevents breakdown of body fat into energy. Insulin stops the enzyme that breaks up triglycerides (fat storage molecules) into fatty acids that our body can use for energy. Furthermore, insulin increases the uptake of glucose from the blood into our fat cells. Glucose in our fat cells is used to make glycerol, one of the building blocks of fat.

On top of this, the glucose/insulin metabolism triggers hunger when glucose is low. This occurs despite an overabundance of fuel that is stored as fat. We are tricked into consuming more glucose to keep this cycle going. The vicious cycle of high carbohydrate/glucose/insulin must be stopped somewhere.

HOW TO STOP GETTING FAT

As we eat less carbohydrates, less glucose is released into the bloodstream, less glucose is stored, and less insulin is needed. If we add high intensity exercise, the stores of glycogen in our muscles will be used. Once the cells are emptied of glycogen, receptors on the cells will become more sensitive to insulin and more efficient at storing glucose. Less insulin is needed to achieve the same result. Once less insulin is present in the bloodstream, fat breakdown will not be inhibited by insulin. This will let us burn more energy stored as fat. A way to accelerate this process is through high intensity interval training (HIIT). This will be covered further in Chapter 5.

There are many low carbohydrate diets available. The best diet is one that is sustainable; it becomes more of a lifestyle than a diet. However, to drastically change your metabolism quickly, we are believers in the power of a ketogenic diet. The process of switching your metabolism from glucose to ketone bodies will transform your body into a fat burning machine.

KETOGENIC DIET

What is a ketogenic diet?

A diet is ketogenic if the body turns fat into ketone bodies and uses that as fuel. There are many ways to achieve this. The most common is a high fat, low carbohydrate diet. It can be summed up as easily as saying a diet consisting of meats, eggs, and green leafy vegetables. Most ketogenic diets call for a ratio of macronutrients of 70% fat, 20% protein, and 10% carbohydrates. This can be tracked simply and easily with an application on your smartphone that logs your food intake for the day. With a ketogenic diet, metabolic transformation takes place, and a person's body goes into ketosis. A ketogenic diet mimics the metabolism when starving. We can use this to trick our body into burning fat.

What is a ketone?

A ketone is a compound that our body can use for energy as an alternative to glucose. The liver makes three ketones, also known as ketone bodies. They are:

- Acetone
- Acetoacetate
- B-Hydroxybutyrate

Though not technically a ketone chemically speaking, B-Hydroxybutyrate (BHB) is able to be metabolized and used like a true ketone. Most commercially available exogenous ketones are a form of B-Hydroxybutyrate.

The most reliable way to find out if you are in ketosis is to measure the level of B-hydroxybutyrate in your blood. Accurate monitors are available for home use and are relatively inexpensive. It is not necessary to continuously test for ketosis if the total carbohydrate count in the diet is kept low. People will respond differently to the switch in their diet and the length of time it takes to get into ketosis will vary from person to person.

By severely limiting carbohydrates, a ketogenic diet may eliminate many of the problems associated with disordered glucose metabolism. Ketone bodies are parts of fatty acids that the body can use for energy. Ketone bodies can be obtained through both exogenous (food or supplements) and endogenous (produced by liver primarily) sources. The goal of a ketogenic diet is to achieve ketosis, a state where ketone bodies are elevated in the blood stream. Many diets (most notably the Atkins Diet) take advantage of this metabolic pathway to accelerate fat burning. There are many other benefits from this approach as well.

The ketogenic diet has been used medically to treat seizure disorders in children that have not responded to medication, reduce tremors in Parkinson's, improve cognition in Alzheimer's, improve the remission rate of cancer treatment, and improve blood sugar and lipid profile in diabetic patients.[18] The key to this is the effect of the ketogenic diet on mitochondria.

Mitochondria are the "power plants" of the cell and are responsible for producing energy. This process normally produces reactive oxygen species, known as free radicals. Free radicals, if left unchecked, can damage our cells. Our bodies have natural defenses in place to quench these free radicals, thereby limiting the damage they can cause. In the presence of a high carbohydrate diet, increased free radical species are present; inflammation is everywhere. Our systems are overwhelmed and inflammation is triggered throughout the body. Inflammation is implicated in many disease processes including heart disease and chronic pain syndromes.

Not only are reactive oxygen species reduced and inflammation decreased with a ketogenic diet, but mitochondria efficiency is improved. Mitochondria generate up to three times more energy by burning ketones compared to glucose. For the nerds, this process is called B-oxidation. High fat, low carbohydrate diets typically provide a robust, steady supply of energy that is protected from the ups and downs of poor glucose metabolism.

BENEFITS OF A KETOGENIC DIET

While some of the benefits of a ketogenic diet have been alluded to above, we felt it would be helpful to explicitly discuss these benefits here. Scientific studies that have shown these benefits are referenced for those interested. A ketogenic diet has been shown to impact, treat, and in some cases reverse disease states in addition to helping to achieve weight loss and looking and feeling better.

Ketogenic diets are an extremely powerful means of providing rapid weight loss. We have seen this time and again in our patients who are attempting to lose weight, and we have seen success where other diets had failed in the past. Compared to low-fat high-carb diets, ketogenic diets produced 2-3 times as much weight loss in randomized controlled trials.[19, 20] Abdominal fat can be decreased on a ketogenic diet by 20% in 12 weeks.[21] Additional studies have shown improvements in weight loss using ketogenic diets versus traditional low-fat or calorie-restricted diets and some studies have shown an increased ability to maintain that weight loss.[22,23]

The second benefit that we would like to highlight is that ketogenic diets have been shown to improve symptoms of depression in some studies.[24,25] Additionally, improved mental clarity has been a touted benefit to a ketogenic diet seen in at least one study.[26] Research overall remains insufficient to determine definitively what effect ketogenic diets have on mental health, but current research findings are promising.

Diabetes is a disease that can cause devastating effects on the lives of those who struggle with it. A significant benefit of the keto diet is that it has been shown to help control blood sugar levels, decrease the dosages needed of diabetic medications, and in some cases to even reverse diabetes.[27-30] Research has been clear that the ketogenic diet can help improve diabetes and decrease insulin resistance when followed properly. Your physician can help to guide you further on how a ketogenic diet can become part of your diabetes treatment.

Although often criticized as a diet that may increase the risk of heart disease, much of the science actually shows that the ketogenic diet likely *reduces* the risk of heart disease. Keto diets have been shown to elevate HDL (good) cholesterol and decrease LDL (bad) cholesterol and triglycerides.[21] These changes are associated with a decreased risk for atherosclerosis and coronary heart disease. Keto diets can also help to reduce the risk of heart disease by causing a decrease in blood pressure.[31] It is important to discuss with your doctor your individual risks for heart disease and how the ketogenic diet may be right for you.

The ketogenic diet has been known to be a successful treatment for epilepsy (seizure disorder) for approximately 100 years. Modern studies confirm this treatment.[32-34] In addition to epilepsy, ketogenic diets have shown potential benefit in other neurological disorders as well.[35-38]

We are not going to make the claim here that ketogenic diets cure cancer, but just know that there are studies which suggest there may be benefits to ketogenic diets in certain types of cancer and many cancer cells heavily rely on glucose for fuel. Ketogenic diets are also highly beneficial for people with certain bowel disorders. Ask your doctor for more information on the benefits of ketogenic diets for disease states.

Benefits of a Ketogenic Diet
▪ Providing and maintaining weight loss
▪ Decreases abdominal fat
▪ Improvement of mental health and clarity
▪ Control blood sugar levels and decrease the need for insulin
▪ Reduce the risk of heart disease
▪ Treatment of diseases such as epilepsy

Table 2.1—Benefits of a Ketogenic Diet

HOW DO I FOLLOW A KETOGENIC DIET?

A ketogenic diet is an answer for anyone struggling with excess body fat. In its simplest form (i.e., don't eat carbs) it is easy to understand and, with proper planning, easy to follow. The initial step in improving the metabolic dysfunction from a high carbohydrate diet is to acclimate the body to burning ketones as an alternative fuel. This process, known as keto-adaptation, can take variable amounts of time depending on your genetic profile. Certain enzymes, cell receptors, and metabolic pathways that have been dormant for years will need to be upregulated in your body. Think about athletic performance as a comparison. Some athletes require months of adaptation before a performance improvement can be seen. Other people can develop skills more quickly. The same goes for your body adaptations to a ketogenic diet.

The first step to transition from glucose to ketones is to stop feeding yourself glucose. This can be done several ways. If you are on a diet consisting almost exclusively of refined carbohydrates, it may be very difficult to transition to a high fat, moderate protein, low carbohydrate diet quickly. Remember, the goal is a sustainable program for continued fat loss. It may be more prudent to gradually decrease the percentage of calories obtained by carbohydrates until the desired amount (less than 20 grams/day) has been reached. For those with strong will power and/or the patience (lack thereof) of a surgeon, a cold turkey approach may work. Another approach is to eat foods only from an approved low carb list.

The goal is to stop eating carbohydrates so that the body is fueled by ketones that we either consume (exogenous) or we produce by burning fat (endogenous). If we eat less glucose, the body will need to produce both glucose and ketone bodies for energy. The body will preferentially burn glucose when it is available, so it is key to decrease the glucose we consume. This will unlock the power of the ketogenic diet.

The first two weeks of this process can trigger symptoms known as the "keto flu." This may be due to electrolyte imbalances and/or dehydration. Symptoms can include fatigue, irritability, dizziness, increased urination, muscle cramps, and constipation. Lovely. The exact reasons for the keto flu are unknown, but it may be accurate to describe it as carbohydrate withdrawal. Ingestion of exogenous ketones (BHB), increased salt and water intake, and ingestion of healthy oils (such as MCT oil) may help to decrease the symptoms of keto flu.

The switch in diet from processed, refined, carbohydrates to a thoughtful one based on real food has not caused consistent, measurable micronutrient deficiencies. This is a concern for long term use, particularly if the diet is not well thought out.

WHAT TO EAT

It will be easiest to only eat foods made from ingredients found in Table 2.2 initially, although this list can expand as time goes on and you build understanding of a ketogenic diet. Many other resources are available as well online to find foods that are appropriate for a ketogenic diet.

Appropriate Foods for a Ketogenic Diet	
Meat of any kind (beef, lamb, etc.)	Avocado
Fish/seafood	Macadamia nuts
Whole eggs	Lemon and lime juice
Sausage	Butter/ghee
Spices and herbs	Heavy cream
Healthy fats (*see left column table 3.1*)	Green leafy vegetables
Low carb protein shakes	Cauliflower
Cheeses	MCT oil

Table 2.2—List of Foods to Eat on a Ketogenic Diet

FASTING

Another way to achieve ketosis is to stop eating. Once available stores of glucose are burned off, the body will turn to fat as a fuel source. This is a way to help your body get into a state of ketosis quickly, and is utilized by some in a technique termed "intermittent fasting," whereby food is eaten for only a specified portion of the day, and during the rest of the day no food is ingested. Intermittent fasting can be accomplished with different programs, but one common and effective way in the beginning to do intermittent fasting is by eating food only within a time period of 8 hours during the day, and fasting for 16, then repeating. Without the intermittent glucose peaks and valleys, the hunger pains that occur from fasting often go away. Health benefits have been reported from intermittent fasting alone, and combined with a ketogenic diet can lead to significant weight loss.

3 | JUST THE FATS

It will be difficult at first to accept how drastically different your diet will be compared to the Standard Western Diet of today. We have been told for years that fat makes us fat. This simply is not true. There is no scientific evidence for this, and it makes little sense metabolically. The culprit, as we have found out, is the sugar-laden diet high in processed carbohydrates. We now, therefore, switch our diet to primarily fat and flip the switch on our metabolism from glucose to ketones.

Saturated fat? Trans fat? What are these terms and what do they mean for our diets and health? We will begin by explaining these and other terms that describe fats.

Fats are made up of chains of carbon, hydrogen, and oxygen molecules. At its core is glycerol alcohol, and three fatty acid chains are attached to this core. Unsaturated fats have double bonds between carbon atoms, while saturated fats have single bonds between carbon atoms. Saturated fats are further described as short, medium, or long-chain based on the length of the fatty acids attached to the core. The length of carbon chains ranges from 2-22.

Long-chain saturated fats (12-18 carbon units in length) are the most efficient energy storage molecule in the body. As such, they constitute the majority of stored fat energy. This is the excess energy we have squirreled away on top of our abs and an important source of fuel as we change our metabolism. Long-chain saturated fats are "clean burning," leaving only carbon dioxide and water as metabolic by-products. They have many benefits including increasing HDL (good cholesterol) and making LDL (the bad cholesterol) less bad by causing them to be less likely to form plaque on arteries.[39]

Foods Rich in Saturated Fat	
Coconut Oil	87%
Dairy	64%
Ground Beef	38%
Egg Yolks	30%

Table 3.1—Food Products Rich in Saturated Fat

Historically, medical advice has encouraged limiting saturated fat intake. Saturated fat is thought to increase cholesterol levels, clogging arteries. The available scientific evidence, however, clearly does not support this. The evidence that does exist shows a weak association, at best. Remember, correlation does not equal causation. More importantly, several studies on low-carb diets have shown improved blood lipid profiles despite higher than recommended saturated fat intake.

Medium-chain saturated fats have, not surprisingly, more medium-sized fatty acids. These medium-chain fatty acids are special because they do not require much digestion and can pass directly to the liver. This allows for a source of energy that can quickly be metabolized. These fats also encourage the development of ketones in the liver. Coconut oil is the primary source for medium-chain saturated fats. Medium-chain triglycerides (MCTs) are worth further discussion.

MCTs are, once again, named based on the length of the carbon chains. C6,8,10,12 (based on the length of the carbon chains) are the most common fatty acids contained in coconut oil. These were named medium by scientists quite arbitrarily. We now know that C12 (lauric acid) is metabolized more like LCTs, meaning that it needs to be processed by the liver prior to use as energy. C12 is the most common MCT found in coconut oil, but the least beneficial metabolically. This is *not* to say that it is unwanted. It has many positive health benefits including antibacterial and antioxidant properties.

True MCTs and their properties that can also be found in coconut oil and can be metabolized quickly include:

C6: Caproic Acid. Bad – can cause throat to burn and generally taste like gasoline. Good – quickly metabolized to ketones. Generally removed from MCT products.

C8: Caprylic Acid. Antimicrobial properties. Fastest metabolized MCT in the brain. Brain Octane Oil.

C10: Capric Acid. More metabolic steps involved to generate energy, but more affordable than C8.

Commercially available MCT products can also be used and can be quickly metabolized to provide energy. Visit www.intelligentcarb.com /supplements to find links to brands that we have used and found to be reputable in our own experience. MCTs are metabolized to ketone bodies. We will discuss direct consumption of ketones (exogenous ketones) later.

Monounsaturated fats are fat molecules where one of the carbon chains contains one double bond within the fatty acid chain. This gives them a higher melting point, so they are generally liquid at room temperature. These fats are universally recognized as "healthy" due to their favorable effects on cardiovascular-disease risk markers. These fats raise HDL, lower LDL and triglycerides, and decrease the amount of oxidized fats and inflammation. Sources of monounsaturated fats include: macadamia nuts, olives, olive oil, avocados, and almonds.

Trans fatty acids are unsaturated fatty acids. Artificial trans fats are implicated in cardiovascular disease and should be avoided. Artificial trans fats are made by partially hydrogenating vegetable oil and have been widely used in the food industry in the past. These fats are present in highly processed snack foods, fried foods, and baked goods. These manufactured fats wreak havoc on blood vessels. They damage the lining and predispose it to plaque formation. LDL is increased with consumption of artificial trans fat. You should make an effort to eliminate all sources of artificial trans fat from your diet faster than a chicken on a junebug. Luckily, artificial trans fats have been banned effective in 2018.

Natural trans fats, on the other hand, are good. Natural trans fats are produced in animals (primarily cows) which consume grass. Grass-fed beef, then, is a good source of this. Conjugated linoleic acid (CLA) is a natural trans fat that has been shown to lower the risk of heart disease, possibly improve insulin sensitivity, reduce the risk of cancer, and reduce body fat. Grass-fed animals contain 3-5 more times conjugated linoleic acid than grain fed animals. Grass-fed beef is certainly more expensive than grain-fed, but based on this might be worthwhile if you can spare the expense. CLA can also be ingested through supplementation. Sources of good trans fats include: dairy products, grass-fed beef, and lamb.

Polyunsaturated fats complicate things even more. We will keep this as simple as possible. Polyunsaturated fats can be divided into two categories: omega-6 and omega-3. They both have important roles in cell structure and regulation. Too much omega-6 and too little omega-3 can contribute to a pro-inflammatory state. There are 2 essential fatty acids that are polyunsaturated fats. These cannot be made by our bodies and must be consumed: Linoleic acid (omega-6), and Alpha-linolenic acid (omega-3).

Linoleic acid is found in small amounts in many foods, particularly nuts, seeds, poultry, and avocados. Importantly, it is also found in large amounts in refined oils (sunflower, corn, soybean). When an excessive amount of linoleic acid is consumed, evidence suggests that it contributes to inflammation. These commercial oils are very cheap and therefore contained in many processed foods such as salad dressings and snacks.

Other omega-6 fats include arachidonic acid, and have been shown to have beneficial effects on health. They are found primarily in animal foods and eggs. These are safe to consume.

The bottom line with omega-6 fats is to **avoid fats from processed oils**.

Alpha-linolenic acid (omega-3) is the other essential fatty acid. It is found in plants. DHA (docosahexaenoic acid) is made from Alpha-linolenic acid (ALA) and could be thought of as a third essential fatty acid, as the metabolic pathway from ALA to DHA is very inefficient. DHA has many health benefits. It is found in phytoplankton, algae, and the animals that eat them. Deficiencies in DHA and EPA (another omega-3) contribute to systemic inflammation and chronic disease. Studies have shown that consumption of omega-3 fatty acids have more substantial effects on cardiovascular health than statins (medications prescribed to help lower high cholesterol).

ALA is primarily found in fruits, vegetables, nuts, and seeds. EPA and DHA are found in greatest concentration in cold water fish such as salmon, mackerel, sardines, tuna, and herring. All three can be ingested through diet or with the use of trusted "fish oil" supplements.

Our human diet over time has shifted away from a 1:1 or 2:1 ratio of omega-6 to omega-3 consumption. Many scientists hypothesize that this change has implications on systemic inflammation and chronic disease.[40] The primary driver of this change is the addition of processed oils.

A case can be made here for eating grass-fed beef, as the omega-6:omega-3 ratio changes from 1.5:1 with grass-fed to 7.7:1 for grain-fed. CLA content, as mentioned earlier, is much higher in grass-fed beef as well. Grain-fed chicken breast has an 18:1 ratio.[41] Similar findings are seen with eggs. Up to 10 times higher omega-3 content is seen in pasture-raised chickens.

Generally, 20 ounces of cold water fish per week will supply the necessary amount of EPA and DHA. Fish oil supplements, while popular and easily accessible, do not all offer the same health benefits. This may be due to processing, subjecting the oils to oxidation. This leads us down the inflammatory pathway, the very thing we hope to avoid. Nutritional supplements are not regulated, and often times obtaining nutrients via whole foods is safer and more predictable. For further information on trusted fish oil supplements, visit www.intelligentcarb.com/supplements.

We realize this has been a lot of information. In summary, we present Table 3.2. Bottom line with fats....

- Saturated and monounsaturated fats should be eaten liberally on a ketogenic diet.
- Avoid processed oils.
- Eat up to 20 ounces of cold water fish weekly

Eat Liberally	Moderate	Never
Coconut oil	Nuts	Soybean oil
Olive oil	Seeds	Peanut oil
Ghee	Nut butters	Corn oil
Butter		Safflower oil
Lard		Canola oil
Duck fat		Sunflower oil
Dairy fat		Grapeseed oil
Eggs		
Meat		
Seafood		

Table 3.2—Fats: What to Eat and What to Avoid

Counting calories is difficult as well as time consuming. Fortunately, on a ketogenic diet there is no need to count calories. Being mindful to include plenty of healthy fats is the biggest tip we can give for beginners on a ketogenic diet.

4 | INTELLIGENT CARB

Now that we have discussed the advantages and concepts of ketogenic diets, we would like to introduce the term "Intelligent Carb." Although we are advocates of a strict ketogenic diet for rapid weight loss and a shift in metabolic health, it can be difficult for some to sustain a pure ketogenic diet over the long term. For some it will be difficult to sustain for even more than a couple of weeks. For this reason, we advocate Intelligent Carb ingestion. As with other ketogenic diets, one central goal in the Intelligent Carb diet is to avoid sugar and spikes in insulin. The large quantities of fat consumption, however, are not required in the Intelligent Carb diet. Additionally, some carbs – Intelligent Carbs – are allowed.

WHAT IS AN INTELLIGENT CARB?

Unlike human beings, all carbs are not created equal. The primary difference to note is between "simple carbohydrates" and "complex carbohydrates." The terms simple and complex refer to the molecular structure of the carbohydrate, and to put it simply, complex carbs are larger molecules than simple carbohydrates. Simple carbs are found in fruits, yogurt, honey, and milk, as well as in processed sugars found in syrups, candy, soda, fruit juices, and table sugar. While most carbohydrates are ultimately digested and enter the bloodstream as glucose, simple carbohydrates are broken down much more quickly than complex carbohydrates. This causes a spike in your blood sugar (serum glucose levels), as described in Chapter 1, and provides a quick supply of energy to fuel your body's cellular functions. This sudden increase in blood sugar leads to the pancreas releasing insulin, which removes sugar from the blood and forces it into your body cells. This results in lower blood sugar levels and makes you feel hungry again. At the same time insulin is being released, the pancreas reduces its production of a substance called glucagon. Glucagon signals to allow stored body fat to be used as energy. Glucagon can, therefore, be thought of as the molecular equivalent of a personal trainer. It is telling your body fat to get up, get moving into the bloodstream and provide energy for your muscles. Glucagon is good in this manner and you want it around enough to help decrease fat stores. Its production is decreased when insulin is increased, and eating simple sugars causes this to happen. It should be noted, however, that glucagon is not all good. In addition to causing the breakdown of fat for energy production it can also lead to the breakdown of muscle, which we want to avoid.

Complex carbohydrates, like simple carbohydrates, are broken down into glucose and enter your bloodstream. Unlike simple sugars, complex carbohydrates take longer to digest and, therefore, when eaten in moderate quantities do not cause the same spike in blood sugar that happens when eating simple carbs. Because they take longer to break down, glucose is more slowly released into the bloodstream. This avoids the necessity to release high amounts of insulin to bring down blood sugar levels.

Complex carbohydrates come from foods such as fresh vegetables, beans, avocados, and almonds (fiber carbs). These foods are rich in fiber, so serve to satisfy hunger and help you feel full. Complex carbs also most often come from foods that are high in vitamins and minerals. However, complex carbs can be found in starchy foods such as pastas, potatoes, brown rice, etc. Unfortunately, a higher starch content can cause more rapid spikes in blood sugar than will high fiber carbs.

As you can see at this point there is not only a distinction between simple and complex carbohydrates, but also between different types of complex carbohydrates (fibers and starches). Glycemic index is a ranking system for foods that is meant to account for this phenomenon of how carbohydrates in foods affect blood sugar levels. Foods with a lower glycemic index cause a slower spike in blood sugar than do foods with a high glycemic index. To put it simply, Intelligent Carbs are those that do not cause rapid, large spikes in blood sugar.

We would like to take a brief pause and note that this is in many ways an oversimplification of a complex topic. It could be debatable whether beans (legumes) get treated as a fiber carb or a starch carb. The same could be said of some other complex carbohydrates as well. The point here is not to get bogged down too much at this stage, but rather to get the idea that most of the carbs you ingest will eventually either get broken down into glucose and absorbed or will be excreted without being digested. The goal is to ingest moderate amounts of Intelligent Carbs – carbohydrates that are filling and are absorbed as slowly as possible or not at all.

Another term that you may hear and read about is "net carbs." Net carbs are calculated by taking the total number of carbohydrates (in grams) from the nutrition label and subtracting the fiber and any sugar alcohols that are present in what you are eating (again in grams).

Net Carbs = Total Carbs – Fiber – Sugar Alcohols

Sugar alcohols are substances such as erythritol, glycerin, mannitol, etc. These substances can produce a sweet taste to food as a substitute for sugar (sucrose). If what you are eating does not have a label, then nutrition facts are available on the internet or through an app on your smartphone.

The reason for calculating net carbs in the first place is that the carbs you are subtracting will often have little or no effect on raising blood sugar. This is because most sugar alcohols are poorly absorbed in the intestine and have a low glycemic index, however, some do have a higher glycemic index (such as Maltitol) and thus may be more capable of raising blood sugar.

Although carbs that come from sugar alcohols are better than those that come from sugar, you should still make an effort to keep these types of carbohydrates to a minimum, as they can cause gastrointestinal problems and the long-term effects of ingesting these substances in large quantities is not completely known. A few examples of how to calculate net carbs are available in figures 4.1-4.3.

Total carbs – Fiber – Sugar Alcohols = Net Carbs
7 g total carbs – 3 g fiber – 0 g sugar alcohols = 4 g net carbs

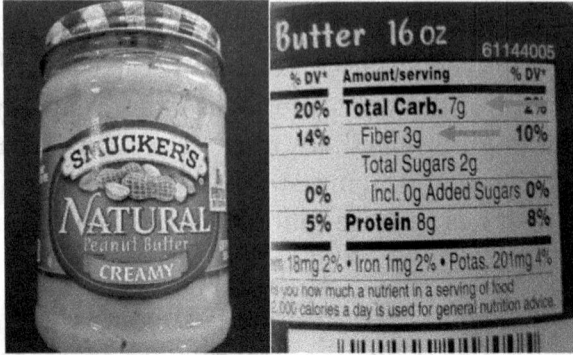

Figure 4.1—Net Carb Calculation for Smucker's Natural Peanut Butter

Total carbs – Fiber – Sugar Alcohols = Net Carbs
6 g total carbs – 3 g fiber – 2 g erythritol = 1 g net carbs

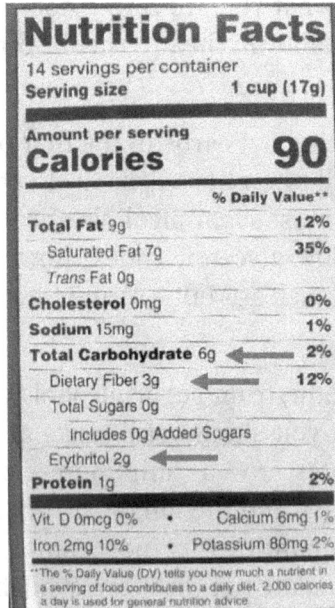

Figure 4.2—Net Carb Calculation for SlimFast Keto Fat Bomb Peanut Butter Cup

Total carbs – Fiber – Sugar Alcohols = Net Carbs
20 g total carbs – **14** g fiber – **2** g glycerin = **4** g net carbs

Amount Per Serving		
Calories 160	**Fat Calories** 80	
		% Daily Value
Total Fat 9g		14%
Saturated Fat 6g		30%
Trans Fat 0g		
Polyunsaturated Fat 0g		
Monounsaturated Fat 2g		
Cholesterol 5mg		2%
Sodium 200mg		8%
Potassium 160mg		5%
Total Carbohydrate 20g ←		7%
Dietary Fiber 14g ←		56%
Sugars 1g		
Glycerin 2g ←		
Protein 10g		17%

Figure 4.3 Net Carb Calculation for Atkins Caramel Double Chocolate Crunch Bar

THE INTELLIGENT CARB DIET

When eating Intelligent Carbs, carbohydrates can be ingested, however, they will come from sources that avoid spikes in blood sugar levels. These carbohydrates will help to make you feel more full and boost your energy. Keeping your carbohydrate intake still relatively low and only from Intelligent Carb sources, you will keep your body primed for fat burning.

There is no need to count carbs, or otherwise perform any complex calculations with your meals. You will not need to count calories, or determine percentages of micronutrients contained in each plate. An eating plan should be simple and straightforward, so that it can and will be followed. As a general rule, you can split your plate (or bowl) into nearly equal thirds and add meat, vegetables, and another Intelligent Carb (avocado, legumes, seeds, nuts) in nearly equal amounts until you have the amount of food you wish to eat. While you can aim for 3 nearly equal sized servings of each meal component, it is perfectly acceptable (and perhaps even preferable) to increase the amount of meat or vegetables and decrease the amount of the second Intelligent Carb chosen with the meal. If you are hungry, you should eat. As long as you are eating approved foods you are all right.

The meat will give you high sources of protein and fats without carbohydrates. The vegetable portion of the meal will provide you with needed vitamins and fiber. A vegetable will make up one of two Intelligent Carbs chosen at every meal. The second Intelligent Carb chosen will be another food which is a low glycemic index food that also contains fiber. These foods have been shown to have an inverse relationship between consumption and incidence of Type II diabetes in adults.[42]

Table 4.1 lists foods that are allowed on the Intelligent Carb diet. This list is not comprehensive but does provide a good variety of Intelligent-Carb-approved foods to get you started. These foods can be mixed and matched to provide an assortment of tastes to make up each meal. In addition to eating different combinations of foods to make up new meals, spices and hot sauces can be added for variety. Just be sure to check prior to using that sauces and dressings contain minimal carbs (2 or 3 g at most) and no sugar (1 g at most). For sauces that contain *any* carbs or sugar, use extremely sparingly.

Meat/Protein	Vegetables	Beans (& the like)
Chicken	Spinach (and other leafy green vegetables)	Black beans
Turkey	Zucchini	Pinto beans
Ground beef	Peppers	Red beans
Fish	Fennel	Lentils
Pork	Broccoli	Refried beans
Canned tuna	Eggplant	Black-eyed peas
Sausage	Green beans	Green Peas
Steak	Cabbage	Split Peas
Eggs	Mushrooms	Lima Beans
	Cauliflower*	Avocado
	Asparagus	Seeds (sunflower, pumpkin)
	Brussel Sprouts	Nuts (macadamia, almond)

Table 4.1—Foods that Can Be Eaten on the Intelligent Carb Diet

Take one or more items from each column. Additional foods can be added that have low net carbs as you get used to eating Intelligent Carbs. Recipes and additional foods can be found in Chapter 7 and at www.intelligentcarb.com.

*Cauliflower can be used as a substitute for several high carb foods such as mashed potatoes, rice, crusts etc.

Shopping can be simplified when following a purely ketogenic or the Intelligent Carb lifestyle. Choose a few meats, vegetables, and other Intelligent Carbs that you enjoy, and stay away from starchy carbs and sugar. Find a few ways to prepare meats and vegetables and mix and match the different meal components to make up many different meal choices. When you add spices and sauces, you have an enormous selection of meals to choose from.

Eat a meal anytime you are hungry. You can aim to eat around every 4-5 hours (unless utilizing intermittent fasting, discussed briefly in Chapter 2). Snacking in between meals is okay, as long as snacks come from Intelligent-Carb-approved foods. Most snacks should be eaten sparingly and some examples can be found in Table 4.2.

All drinks should be free of calories and carbohydrates with some exceptions: low carbohydrate protein shakes are okay to drink either as meal supplements, meal replacements, or snacks. Protein drinks should be high in protein, low in carbs (2-3 net per serving), and low or no sugar (1 g or less). Water with lemon or unsweetened iced tea can and should be consumed with every meal and snack.

Avoid drinks with artificial sweeteners or at least use sparingly (no more than one diet soft drink per day, and even that is probably too much).

Coffee is certainly okay to drink as well but avoid any creamers that contain sugars and avoid artificial sweeteners in coffee as well. Heavy cream, coconut oil, butter, vanilla extract, and cinnamon can all be added to coffee if desired.

Snacks
Small handful of almonds
Brazil nuts
Macadamia nuts
Pistachios
Garbanzo beans
Beef jerky (rarely, and only low-in-sugar brands/flavors)
Slice of turkey wrapped around sliced cucumber with cream cheese spread
Salad with vinaigrette, mayonnaise, or other low-carb dressing with no processed oils
Cheese (especially Brie, cheddar, Colby jack, Monterey jack, parmesan, blue cheese, goat cheese)
Artichoke
Almond milk
Buffalo chicken dip
Celery (and other raw low-carb vegetables)
Pork rinds
Avocado with crushed macadamia nuts and MCT oil

Table 4.2—Example Snacks that Can Be Eaten in Small Quantities

WHAT YOU SHOULDN'T EAT

Now that you have a plentiful list of foods you can eat, it may be helpful to briefly discuss foods that are not part of an Intelligent Carb diet. A good general rule to use that is easy to fall back on (if you forget all else) is simply to avoid foods that are white. For example, potatoes, rice, bread, pasta – are all starch carbs with a high glycemic index that will spike your blood sugar and should be avoided, except during a cheat meal (which will be discussed soon).

If you find yourself unsure about whether a food with carbs can be eaten, look to make sure it is low in sugar, and has at least half as many grams of fiber as it has grams of carbs. If it does, then it is most probably okay to have in small quantities from time to time. Otherwise you can go to our website at www.intelligentcarb.com/glycemicindex and find links to sites where you can tell whether a food has a low or a high glycemic index. In general, foods with a GI over 55 are considered to have a high glycemic index and should be avoided.

In addition to avoiding the above foods, we would also recommend avoiding certain drinks. Diet soda, while it may mimic the taste of regular soda without adding calories, seems to be detrimental to weight loss. The exact mechanism of this is not clear yet, but there is a dose-response (higher dose gives a bigger response) relationship between diet soda and abdominal obesity.[43] Drink plenty of water. Feel free to add lemon or lime juice. We enjoy sparkling water as well.

MEAL PREPARATION FOR THOSE WHO THINK THEY CAN'T (OR DON'T LIKE TO) COOK

We have both heard the following excuses many times from people: "I don't like to cook," or "I can't cook, and therefore I have a hard time sticking with a diet." Another common excuse is, "I'm too busy to prepare healthy food." If you have ever used any of these phrases or made some similar statement, then this section is for you.

You do not have to be a professional chef (or really have any skill at all in the kitchen) to follow a successful Intelligent Carb diet. You may need to occasionally turn on the oven or the stove once in a while (we know this is an unfamiliar concept for some people reading this), but believe us, it's not that hard to do once you try it. Most times a microwave will be the most complex appliance you will be using. A barbeque, slow cooker, or portable grill can take the place of the oven if it must.

There are many types of meat (proteins) that are acceptable on an Intelligent Carb eating program. Chicken, fish, hamburgers, etc., can all be purchased at relatively inexpensive prices, stored for several months, and cooked with little effort in large enough quantities to last for several days.

Preparation can be as simple as turning on the oven to the appropriate temperature, placing the meat on an oven pan (you can lay down tinfoil to make clean-up easier), and setting a timer while it cooks. Even if you don't "cook," you can do this. If however, you determine that this is still too much cooking for you, there are other options. If you like to barbeque you can take the meat you wish to prepare for the next several days and cook it on the grill, then save it for later to be reheated in the microwave. If you cook on your cheat day (see the last section of this chapter), you can even enjoy a cold beer while you do it.

Other options for cooking meat with minimal effort include slow-cooker recipes using low carb ingredients and pre-prepared meals in the frozen section that are low/no carb that you just open and heat up on a stovetop (such as frozen fajita packages, etc.). Leftovers from these meals can usually be stored well and remain fresh for several days for quick meals that require reheating only in the microwave.

Eggs are another source of healthy fat and protein for your meals that can be prepared simply. We recommend having hard-boiled eggs available in the refrigerator to eat for breakfast on the go, as a snack, or to add extra protein to salads/other meals. Scrambled eggs can even be prepared in the microwave in just a few minutes by simply beating the eggs in a microwave safe bowl, heat for 45 seconds, stir, and heat another 30 seconds. Sausage goes great with eggs and is another meat that can be cooked easily.

Beans can come from a can, so your preparation can be as easy as opening the can and heating the beans in a bowl using the microwave. While there is nothing wrong with making beans this way, we find it convenient to periodically make large batches using dried beans from a bag, then at mealtime heat up a scoop. A recipe for beans can be found in Chapter 7.

Finally, vegetable preparation can be done quickly and simply by filling a bowl with spinach, covering, placing in the microwave and cooking as desired. Spinach, and other vegetables can also be added to a meal raw. A salad with low carb dressing can be added to a meal, or can be the meal itself as long as it contains a good source of protein. Finally, precut and seasoned vegetables can be purchased at most supermarkets that require simply cooking in some healthy oil (MCT, olive, etc.) on the stove, in the oven, or in the microwave for a couple minutes.

Hopefully this section has gotten rid of your last possible excuse as to why you cannot eat healthy food. You don't have to spend a lot of time to prepare healthy meals – in fact, healthy meals can be prepared in less time than it takes to get in your car and go through the drive-thru at your favorite fast-food restaurant, and you don't have to be a great chef to do it. But who knows, start cooking simple things, add your own tricks and flare, and you may even become one.

EATING OUT

Many people find eating out to be a major contributing factor to diet failure. This is unfortunate given that eating out provides social interaction, a break from routine meals at home, and a chance to experience new ways to prepare foods. Eating out is fun and enjoyable to most people, but unfortunately for many, they must choose between eating out or sticking to their diet. Fortunately, this is rarely if ever a problem for someone living the Intelligent Carb lifestyle.

When out at a restaurant, continue to keep things simple in choosing what to eat (just like you do when you're at home). Choose whatever type of meat you are in the mood for and add sides such as those found in Table 4.1. Avoid appetizers (for the most part) and try a small salad instead with a vinaigrette dressing. Avoid dessert at the end of the meal as well. Ask your server to substitute vegetables for potatoes, or simply don't eat the potatoes (or other high carb food) when they are served to you.

Just because a certain food is served to you does not mean you must eat it. When you're out at a restaurant it is not the same as it was when you sat at your mother's dinner table: you do not have to clean your plate before you get up from the table. You are not going to offend anyone by not eating the food they toiled over to prepare for you. You will disappoint yourself, however, by having lost your willpower when you do eat those high carb foods.

Another solution to the eating out issue is to try to time eating out with a day where you have planned to have your cheat meal. Many restaurants today have specific keto-friendly menu options as well.

Several fast-food restaurants can accommodate Intelligent Carb meals as well. Most restaurants that sell hamburgers will do so without the bun, either in a bowl or wrapped in a piece of lettuce. You can even double the meat or cheese and add bacon. Grilled chicken is also abundantly available in fast-food settings. There will probably be some fast-food restaurants that you will just need to avoid altogether (except when you go for a cheat meal), but feel free to get creative here. Low carb lifestyles are accommodated by most restaurants.

ALCOHOL

Alcohol should be used sparingly, for the most part, but does not need to be cut out altogether. A night of heavy drinking, however, will kick you out of ketosis and may increase your fat stores. Most types of straight, unflavored spirits such as bourbon, vodka, rum, gin, etc., contain no carbohydrates and can be used in moderation on an Intelligent Carb diet. Served on the rocks or neat, with a twist of lemon or lime, or garnished with a cucumber or celery, straight liquor is a good low carb way to ingest your alcohol. Flavored waters and no-calorie sports drinks work well as mixers.

Beer should be avoided as much as possible during a normal week, however a low carb beer from time to time can be okay (but be careful because these carbs add up; no more than one in a day).

Wine should also be consumed sparingly during a normal week, however one glass of a dry wine (high tannins, often lower sugar, more antioxidants) such as a cabernet sauvignon, merlot, or a dry pinot grigio can be enjoyed from time to time.

It's okay to get creative in moderation with alcohol consumption. For example, one incredibly easy recipe for an Intelligent Carb and delightfully refreshing Moscow Mule is made over ice, filling half of the cup with vodka, the other half with a zero-carb diet ginger beer, and finishing off with a wedge of lime.

ONE MORE THING (CHEAT MEALS)

If you are a human being, you will sometimes get cravings for foods that are not part of your eating plan, often foods that will cause your blood sugar to spike and that will contribute to your weight gain. If you give into these cravings at the wrong times and often enough you can destroy your efforts in no time. Few people have the ability to ignore these cravings completely over the long term without a strategy. This is extremely important, because as a point of fact, even small cheats (a couple of potato chips or a bowl of rice here or there) at the wrong times or with the wrong frequency can completely derail this diet.

Fortunately, there is a relatively easy, minimal harm way you can manage these cravings. By allowing yourself specific times where you eat these foods (in reasonable quantities) you can satisfy your cravings while mitigating the damage these foods can cause. One half-day per week, you can eat a meal and some snacks where you can give into all of your cravings from the week. By having these scheduled cheat meals, you can control your cravings. Rather than telling yourself "no I can't have that," you can tell yourself "I can have that, but I have to wait until Saturday" (or whatever day you choose for your cheat meals). In this manner, you are not depriving yourself of the high carb foods you enjoy, rather you are reinforcing to yourself that there is no need to break your diet; you can have those cookies you crave, just have them on the right day.

We want to state the obvious here – if you follow an Intelligent Carb diet without eating cheat meals, of course you will progress faster on your journey to good health. Especially if trying to lose weight for serious health concerns, you may not want to use cheat days in the beginning. The key here is how long you can strictly follow this or any other diet without built-in cheat meals. If you can completely cut the sugar and starch out of your diet for good – go for it. If you are dieting to improve a medical condition such as diabetes, even infrequent large spikes in blood sugar from these foods can be detrimental. If allowing yourself these cheat meals is the only way you can assure yourself that you will strictly follow a healthier eating plan, however, then the downside is worth it for the overall benefit.

Cheat meals will take you out of ketosis and should be used with caution during a pure ketogenic diet state, as described in Chapter 2, as it will turn off your fat burning for fuel and it can take days to get back into ketosis.

A word of caution regarding cheat meals: although the entire point of the cheat meals is to allow yourself to give in to your food desires and enjoy your meals, use some common sense about it. It is not a day to go on an all-out binge eating spree. For example, eating a 4,000+

calorie meal on your cheat day would be more than a little excessive. In other words, a slice of cheesecake is okay, eating an entire cheesecake – not so much. An interesting phenomenon that we have observed is that the first few bites of a food you have been wanting will completely satisfy the craving, and the remainder is excess calories with little additional benefit.

Feel free to eat a few slices of your favorite pizza, a sandwich, a bowl of cereal, your favorite dessert, etc., but do not eat enough of these items to induce a food coma. It's okay though to go to your favorite fast-food restaurant and get your favorite meal. Have a couple of your favorite cookies crumbled on top of a bowl of ice cream. On the other hand, don't eat an entire box of your favorite cookie. Don't eat an entire large pepperoni pizza. The point is, you want to have enough of what you desire to keep you motivated and on track the rest of the week, but not so much that you erase your entire week's gains.

A good strategy for cheat meals is to plan out those meals ahead of time. As cravings come up during the week, write them down so that you can fulfill those desires on cheat day. Plan out quantities of foods that you will eat for each meal and make sure that you do not leave any leftovers in your refrigerator that will tempt you during the week. Plan to exercise that day, and plan to perform resistance exercises for large muscle groups such as squats or pull-ups. Eat high-protein and low carbohydrate foods as well that day with your cheat foods to keep yourself from overeating the bad stuff.

One additional strategy for cheat day that can be helpful to avoid erasing too much of your hard-earned gains from the week is to wait until noon on your cheat day to begin eating. Eat an Intelligent Carb dinner the night before by 7:00 P.M. and when you wake up the next morning drink plenty of water with lemon in it, and if you are a coffee or tea drinker, go ahead and have that too. Wait to eat anything until at least noon or later, then eat something sensible. After that, have your cheat day consisting of one cheat meal and some snacks. Finish eating on your cheat day by around 8:00 P.M. and avoid eating anything again the following morning until noon. If not eating first thing in the morning is not an option for you, consider eating only high protein and low fat/low carb food (such as egg whites) until you begin your cheat meal(s).

5 | EFFICIENT EXERCISE

From the outset we want to say that some of our favorite exercises to recommend to patients are low impact forms of aerobic exercise. These include activities such as biking, swimming, and using an elliptical trainer. These types of exercise have health benefits way beyond losing weight and looking better. Additionally, strength training can add an important component to an exercise regimen that will help to achieve the goal of getting healthy.

There are many health benefits to gaining muscle. First and foremost, muscle mass supports a higher metabolism. That means that if your body contains a higher percentage of muscle, you will burn more calories at rest than if your body contains a lower percentage of muscle. You can use this to your advantage by targeting a few large muscle groups to exercise in an effort to increase muscle mass with the long-term goal of losing adipose tissue (fat). For most people who are not routine weightlifters already, very significant gains can be made in this area with very little time devoted to it.

Another benefit to muscle strengthening is the protective effect that it can have on your joints. Muscle strengthening in a balanced manner can improve stability in a joint and decrease abnormal stresses. Strengthening for this purpose also goes hand in hand with stretching, and flexibility can be an important component to achieving overall good health (especially in terms of low back health).

An additional benefit to muscle strengthening through resistance training is its effect on bone health. When you expose your bones to increased loads they respond by increasing in density. This can be protective against osteoporosis (brittle bones) and fractures from low energy mechanisms (see Chapter 6).

We would like to address a commonly held myth about strength training. Many people – especially women – avoid strength training altogether because of the belief that by picking up a dumbbell they will become as muscular as the weightlifters on the cover of a bodybuilding magazine. We would like to unequivocally assure you that getting big and muscular like that will never just happen from doing a few resistance exercises here and there. Developing a body like that takes tremendous amounts of time, dedication, and planning. An additional point on this subject is that muscle mass is built up slowly enough that the moment you started to feel that your muscles were getting too big you could back off on your resistance training and your muscles would quickly stop getting bigger, or even atrophy (get smaller). Finally, the exercises described in this chapter are designed more toward increasing muscle strength and endurance, rather than to turn you into a massive bodybuilder.

GETTING STARTED

If you have never done resistance training before, it is important to seek guidance from your physician who knows your individual situation and can guide you in this process. After discussion with your physician, this chapter will help you to begin to develop an exercise routine. If you have limited time available for exercise, the routines in this chapter will provide you with the benefits of strength training in an extremely small amount of time. Finally, if you normally devote hours per day to the gym, we congratulate you on your efforts and realize that you may not have much need for this chapter. However, we encourage you to read this chapter anyway for two reasons: 1) you may occasionally find yourself without a gym (traveling, time constraints, etc.) where you can use one of these workouts to substitute for your typical workout, and 2) because you may know someone (a family member, a friend, or a work colleague) who is not ready for the high level athletic workout you do but would benefit from a little more exercise and you can share these workouts with them.

Your body is designed to adapt to many stresses placed upon it by your environment. When your body's skeletal muscle is stressed (by lifting weights heavier than it is capable of lifting), over time it will adapt by increasing in size in response to these stresses. Muscles can be stimulated to grow by performing an exercise until that muscle group can no longer lift the weight (failure). The last repetition (rep) where you can no longer lift the weight can be referred to as the failure rep. This failure rep is the key to stimulating muscle growth, whether it occurs in the first set you do or in the tenth. We don't want to oversimplify things too much, and there are certainly benefits of doing more sets than one to work a muscle group, but the point here is that efficient and productive workouts can be performed in a limited amount of time. In general, these "efficiency workouts" can be done in 5 minutes or less by choosing one exercise for the body part you are working and doing one quick warm-up set (about 6 reps), and then doing a set to failure (STF).

Concentrate on maximal contraction possible by that muscle as you perform that exercise. On the last rep (failure rep), push/pull/work/strain as hard as you possibly can (with perfect form), flexing the muscle you are trying to work, and continue with maximal effort for a minimum of 7 seconds without any positive movement before counting that as your failure rep. By doing this you have exhausted the muscle(s) involved in the movement you are performing and are stimulating growth.

For these workouts to produce results, it is important you are working your muscles to the *true* point of failure, not just to the point where you *think* your muscles have failed (in other words, you need to achieve muscular failure, not mental failure). This is why we recommend maximal effort for 7 seconds without any positive movement as your indication that you have properly performed a STF. Next, we can look at some specific exercises that can be employed.

EXERCISES

Many of these exercises can be performed with slight variations if desired to work muscle groups slightly differently or to accommodate injuries. While some equipment will be necessary, most of these exercises can be performed without it and can easily be performed while traveling as well. The two recommended pieces of equipment for a beginner to keep expenses low while allowing a complete workout are a pull-up bar and resistance bands. (Visit the website for more information: www.intelligentcarb.com/exercise.)

Pull-ups

Pull-ups are one of the fundamental movements for developing muscle mass. Don't worry if you have never been able to do a pull-up in your life – it's okay, you can still do this. You may need to modify things a bit, but that's all right. A permanent pull-up bar can be installed or one that goes in a doorway and is removable works well too. Again, this is one of the few pieces of equipment you may need to buy if you don't already have one. It is well worth the expense, however.

It is also okay to get creative and use other objects that you can safely hang from to do pull-ups. Many parks have pull-up bars as well. A very good and inexpensive pull-up bar can be made out of a short piece of 1" iron pipe wrapped in tape. If you are unable to perform regular pull-ups on your own, a chair can be placed 1-2 feet in front of you and your feet can go on this chair to allow you to push up with your legs slightly as you pull up with your arms to bring your chin higher than the bar. Control your body on the way down and slowly lower yourself. Your grip should be slightly wider than shoulder width and your palms facing away from you. With pull-ups, try to aim for 20 total reps as your workout (with or without use of the chair and your legs) making sure that you perform one STF. If you find difficulty with your grip (holding onto the bar), straps or gloves can be purchased to assist with grip. With practice hanging and holding onto the bar, grip strength will increase.

Push-ups

Push-ups are another fundamental movement. In the beginning, it is okay to perform push-ups with your knees in contact with the ground, and work your way up to doing traditional push-ups. For people with wrist problems, push-up bars or doing knuckle push-ups (using the business end of your clenched fist as your push-up platform rather than your palm) can help tremendously. Do one warm-up set, rest for about 1 minute, then do one set to failure. As you get stronger, there are many modifications that can be done with push-ups to increase the intensity of the workout, and to introduce slight variations in the manner in which the muscles are worked. For example, push-ups can be performed with a clap, with varied hand positions, with pushing the entire body up and off the floor with arms outstretched with each rep (superman), etc.

Bicep curls

A third exercise that can be incorporated is bicep curls. These can be performed with dumbbells, kettlebells, barbells, bands, etc. It's okay to change your grip at times to add variety to the workouts. Palm up (pointed forward with arms at your side, i.e., supinated) is one common technique to use when performing this exercise and helps to maximally engage the biceps brachii muscle. Keeping your upper arm still and tight against your side, and with palm up, bend at your elbow through a full range of motion from straight to fully bent. The curl can also be performed with palms facing downward, inward, or twisting during the movement. One warm-up set of approximately 10 reps should be performed using around 50% of the weight you will use for your STF. Rest 1 minute, then perform a STF aiming for a weight you can lift for 12-16 reps.

Dips

Dips are another exercise that can be a part of this minimalistic yet highly efficient routine. If you have access to a dip bar and can do at least 10 dips, then by all means dips can be done in that way. You may even add weights to yourself by attaching weights to a belt. If you do not have access to a standard dip station, or if you are a beginner and unable to perform standard dips, a chair is a simple piece of equipment that will allow you to still get a great dip workout. Start seated in the chair with your hands at the edge of the chair, about shoulder width. You can vary your grip with your forearms facing backward (pronated) and your hands on the front edge of the chair, or with your hands on the side edges of the chair with forearms facing each other. Your feet can be kept flat on the floor in front of you with knees bent. Lower yourself down with your arms by bending at the elbows until your upper arms are parallel to the floor. Next, push back up until your elbows are fully extended (arms straight). That is one rep. Perform one warm-up set and one STF.

By straightening your legs further out in front of you, the difficulty level of the exercise goes up. By placing your feet up on a second chair, the difficulty level is further increased. As you advance with this exercise you can try variations such as raising one foot as high as you can in the air or adding weight on your lap.

Squats

Squats (another fundamental exercise for developing muscle mass) can be performed with or without weights. Stand with your back straight, looking forward. Bend at your hips and your knees to 45 degrees (90 degrees if you are without any hip or knee problems and have strong leg muscles), then straighten back up. Aim for 60-90 reps, 1 set. Isometric sets can be done as an alternative. To do this, assume the bottom position of the rep and hold it for as long as you can. The next time try to hold it for longer. As you are able to go lower on this exercise, do so until you can do your reps with your thighs parallel to the floor at the bottom of your reps.

Core training

Core training (such as planks, abdominal crunches, leg raises, seated knee tucks, etc.) can be done periodically (1-2 times per week) as your only exercise for the day or in addition to one of the previously mentioned exercises.

Planks are great to build core strength. Perform these by getting in "push-up position," taking care to maintain a straight line from your shoulders to your toes. You can also rest on your forearms and bend your elbows to 90 degrees for your planks.

Crunches are performed by laying on your back and raising your head and shoulder blades up, holding for a count of two, then slowly lowering back down. Your feet can be on the ground or up in the air.

Leg raises are performed lying flat with feet straight out. Keeping your knees straight, raise your feet six inches off the floor. This is the starting position. Next, raise your feet up until they are about 70 degrees to the ground, then lower back to six inches from the floor and repeat.

A more difficult exercise is called hollow body. Lying flat on your back, your arms should extend overhead while raising your shoulders a few inches off the ground and extending your legs to around 30 degrees off the floor. Hold for as long as you can. Make sure your lower back is in contact with the ground at all times.

Seated knee tucks are performed by sitting on the edge of a bench or a chair. Lean back 45 degrees while holding onto the chair with your feet pointed out in front of you (your body in a straight line). Next, tuck your knees up to your chest then extend back to the starting position and repeat.

Perhaps the easiest core exercise in this workout (especially for beginners) is to perform abdominal crunches from the floor or on an exercise ball for your abdominal work. Forcibly contract when raising up. Try to perform between 20 and 50 reps for one set.

Kettlebell exercises

Kettlebell exercises can also be incorporated into this routine. Any day where a little extra workout is desired, pick a kettlebell exercise. Kettlebell swings are recommended when you are beginning, and then you can work your way up to more difficult kettlebell exercises.

With your feet shoulder width apart, hold the kettlebell between your legs. Keeping your back straight and your arms straight through the entire movement, squat down 45 degrees, allowing weight to swing slightly backward between your legs, then swing the weight up to shoulder level while extending your hips and knees straight, then lower back down. Concentrate on forcefully and explosively pushing your knees back and your pelvis forward during each rep. Start with little (10-20 lbs.) or no weight to get your form down at first. Once you have mastered the movement, move up to using 30-50 lbs., and aim for 60 reps.

2-PHASE APPROACH

Tables 5.1 and 5.2 contain the two phases of this exercise routine. They are similar in their approach to short, efficient workouts, with the main difference being adding an additional set in Phase 2. There is no set time interval where Phase 1 should be performed before moving on to Phase 2, and in fact even after moving on to Phase 2 there is nothing at all wrong with going back to a Phase 1 workout from time to time.

Even after transitioning to more advanced routines that you hopefully will eventually create on your own, there may be occasions where you will want to avoid overtraining or save time by switching back to these efficiency workouts.

Phase 1

Day	Body Part	Exercise	Comments
Saturday	Back	Pull-ups	20 reps total (use chair if needed)
Sunday	Chest	Push-ups	1 STF. Aim for 20-40 reps. OK to modify (from knees, standard, with clap, with weights, etc.)
Monday	Total body conditioning	Interval run	100-yard dash at maximal speed 5-10 times, with 1-2 min walking in between each sprint
Tuesday	Biceps	Bicep curls	1 STF. Pick weight aiming for 12-16 reps
Wednesday	Triceps	Dips	1 STF. Any variation. Aim for at least 12 reps but OK to do up to 40-50 if able. Add weight if needed.
Thursday	Legs	Squats	60-90 reps (no weight). Perform an isometric squat on last rep for as long as you can hold it.
Friday	Recovery/ Total body	Recovery/ Kettlebell exercise	Take this day off as a rest or perform a total body kettlebell exercise such as kettlebell swings, snatch, Turkish get-up, etc.

Table 5.1—Phase I Exercise Program. This program (and the others) can start on any day desired, however we recommend performing a large muscle group exercise (back, chest, legs) on your cheat day.

Phase 2

Day	Body Part	Exercise(s)	Comments
Saturday	Back	Pull-ups (regular and wide grip)	20 reps total regular + 1 set wide grip
Sunday	Chest	Push-ups (regular and decline)	1 STF, + 1 set decline
Monday	Total body conditioning	Interval run, kettlebell exercise	100-yard dash maximal speed 5-10 times, 1-2 min walking in between each sprint, total body kettlebell exercise
Tuesday	Biceps	Bicep curls (palm up and hammer)	1 STF palm up, 1 STF hammer curls
Wednesday	Triceps	Tricep extensions, dips	1 set extensions 12-16 reps each hand, 1 STF dips
Thursday	Legs	Squats, calf raises	60-90 reps squats with isometric last rep, calf raises 40-50 reps with isometric last rep
Friday	Rest/Total body	Rest/Kettlebell exercises	Day off or total body kettlebell exercise

Table 5. 2—Phase II Exercise Program

Additional exercises can be performed that have not yet been mentioned. These exercises can be done as an alternative to those already mentioned, or occasionally one or two of the additional exercises may be performed in conjunction with an exercise of the same body part being worked on the same day. Table 4.3 lists these exercises and the primary body part targeted by each one. A description of these exercises can be found online at www.intelligentcarb/exercise.

Muscle Group	Exercises
Back	Pull-ups, chin-ups, bent row, lat pull-downs, seated row
Chest	Push-ups, bench press, dumbbell press, incline press
Legs	Squats, leg press, calf raises, lunges, dead lift
Shoulders	Military press, shoulder flys, shrugs, upright row
Biceps	Curls (many variations)
Triceps	Dips, tricep extensions, tricep presses, nosebreakers
Core/Abdominals	Crunches, leg lifts, bicycles, ab twists, seated knee tucks, hanging knee raise
Total Body	Kettlebell swings, snatches, power-clean, Turkish get-up

Table 4.3—Exercises that Work Primarily with a Muscle Group. For complete descriptions of each exercise visit www.intelligentcarb.com/exercise.

While the routines in Table 5.1 and Table 5.2 can be used for as long as you may like as your resistance workout, there may be occasions where you have a little more time and want to perform a slightly more intense workout, and have access to gym equipment. In these times, efficient workouts can still be performed by using supersets (performing two exercises back-to-back without rest) and then resting no more than 2 minutes in between each superset. Table 5.4 lists these routines.

Phase 3

Day	Body Part	Exercises	Sets/Reps
Saturday	Back and Biceps (approx. 20 min)	1) Pull-ups 2) Seated rows 2) Curls 3) Lat pull downs behind the head 3) Hammer curls	20 reps total 3 sets: 16, 12, 8 3 sets: 16, 12, 8 2 sets: 16, 12 2 sets: 16, 12
Sunday	Chest and Triceps (approx. 27 min)	1) (Dumbell) Bench press 1) Close grip push-ups 2) Incline press 2) Tricep extensions 3) Incline push ups 3) Dips 4) Chest flys	3 sets: 12, 10, 8 3 sets: aim for 12-20 or more each set 2 sets: 12, 10 2 sets: 16, 12 2 sets: aim for 12-20 or more each set 2 sets: 10-20 reps per set 2 sets: 12, 12
Monday	Total body conditioning	Interval run, kettlebell exercise	100-yard dash maximal speed 5-10 times, 1-2 min walking in between each sprint, total body kettlebell exercise
Tuesday	Shoulders and Legs (approx. 21 min)	1) Shoulder raises 1) Squats 2) Upright rows 2) Calf raises 3) Shrugs	2 sets: 12, 12 2 sets: 60-90 reps + isometric final rep 2 sets: 12, 12 2 sets: 40-50 reps + isometric final rep 2 sets: 20, 20

Wednesday	Total body and Abs (approx. 22 min)	1) Kettlebell swings 1) Abdominal crunches 2) Turkish get-ups 2) Seated knee tucks	2 sets: 50, 50 2 sets: 50, 50 2 sets each side: 20 reps per side, per set 2 sets: 20, 20
Thursday	Rest	Rest	Rest
Friday	Rest	Rest	Rest

Table 5.4—Phase III Exercise Program. Maximum efficiency is gained from performing supersets to work multiple muscle groups in the same day in minimal time.

HIGH INTENSITY INTERVAL TRAINING (HIIT)

High intensity interval training (HIIT) is a category of exercise routines that focus on short, maximal or near maximal bursts of energy (80% or more of maximal heart rate, Table 5.5), combined with short rest periods or low-intensity intervals (for example, a comfortable walking pace). Because of the high intensity nature of this type of exercise, it is important to speak with your doctor prior to beginning a HIIT program to ensure that you are healthy enough to participate. If you have a heart condition, HIIT is likely not for you.

HIIT is an extremely efficient technique of training designed to make the most out of a short available time period. HIIT requires a greater energy expenditure during the workout, but also has the added benefit of helping to burn more calories after the workout when compared to standard aerobic exercise.[44,45] This is because oxygen consumption is significantly increased both during and after exercise with HIIT. That leads to an increased metabolic rate, and ultimately a better waistline. According to the American College of Sports Medicine, benefits of HIIT include improved fitness, blood pressure, insulin sensitivity, body weight, cardiovascular health, and cholesterol profiles. With all those benefits, why wouldn't you devote time to HIIT?

Age	Target Heart Rate (80-100%)	Max Heart Rate (220-age)
20	160-200	200
25	156-195	195
30	152-190	190
35	148-185	185
40	144-180	180
45	140-175	175
50	136-170	170
55	132-165	165
60	128-160	160
65	124-155	155
70	120-150	150
75	116-145	145

Table 5.5—Target Heart Rate for Interval Training Based on Age

A HIIT workout can last anywhere from 5 minutes up to around 40 minutes. It can involve running, jumping, cycling, swimming, etc. The key is having both the high intensity intervals (maximal effort reaching target heart rates) followed by low intensity intervals. These low intensity intervals are essential because they allow your body to return repeatedly to the same maximal high energy expenditure level.

A typical HIIT workout might have 5 cycles of high intensity to low intensity, for example, with 1-minute all-out sprints followed by 1-minute walks for a total of 10 minutes of exercise. There are many types of HIIT workouts that can be performed. Another example would be to jump rope at maximum speed for 30 seconds, rest for 10 seconds, and repeat this cycle 8 times for a workout that lasts just over 5 minutes. It is okay to be creative and come up with your own HIIT workouts as well as long as you follow the general guidelines of high intensity followed by low intensity. For more HIIT workouts, visit www.intelligentcarb.com/exercise.

WORKING OUT AT WORK

Studies have shown that productivity and efficiency for people with sedentary jobs is improved when some form of physical activity is performed during the workday.[46,47] Even brief isometric muscular contractions can stress muscles enough to get blood flowing and can even stimulate muscle growth. Additionally, physical activity has been shown to improve cognition and mood.[48,49]

Relatively few people, however, have access to a gym at their office or are allotted time within their workday to get a 20-30 minute workout done. So what can the average person do to get some kind of workout done and to reap the benefits during the workday? The best advice we can give is first to be creative. You know your individual job responsibilities and your typical day better than anybody. Think about your job and what unique opportunities you have to get exercise done throughout your day.

Can you take stairs instead of an elevator? If so, take as many flights of stairs throughout the day as you can handle, and as you get in better shape, take more. Are you on the telephone a lot during the day? You could get a headset that allows you to get up and walk around while you are on the phone. That will not only give you some exercise while on the phone but you will find that it helps you think and speak better during your telephone conversation. Is there a place at work you can hang from to do pull-ups for a set or two? Perform a set or two of push-ups. If you have occasions at work to go from one building to another within walking distance, make sure that you are walking and not driving. You get the idea at this point, but really think about your specific situation and take advantage of exercising whenever you can.

In addition to getting creative and moving more throughout the day, we recommend performing isometric exercises while at work if that is the only time you can get your workout done. Especially for people who do not regularly lift weights, isometric exercises are a great introduction to muscle training and can provide a good muscle workout for novice weightlifters.

ISOMETRIC TRAINING

Isometric training is beneficial for many reasons, among which are that you can rigorously work your muscles without working up much of a sweat, and you can do this in an extremely short amount of time. In fact, the following workouts at work can be done in under 1 minute, and can be repeated a few times during the day if desired. This is not to say that an isometric workout for 1 minute is going to get you the same results as lifting weights for an hour every day. Isometric training is not going to get you a massive physique. However, it will allow you to get some muscle training done even on days where you lack time. Isometric training also has the benefit of working muscles without movement of the corresponding joints which can have benefit for people with degenerative joint disease (arthritis), in that an isometric workout will stress the involved muscles without causing the grinding that can aggravate joint pain.

Isometric exercises are, in effect, exercises performed by flexing the involved muscle(s) without movement (i.e., the length of the muscle does not change during the exercise). In order to get benefit from isometric training, it is important to flex the targeted muscle with maximal, focused effort for a specified period of time. In the beginning, perform each exercise by putting the muscle under maximal tension for at least 7-10 seconds at a time. Most of the following exercises can all be performed in a chair while sitting at a desk.

Back

To isometrically work the muscles in your back, pull your shoulders back and concentrate on squeezing your shoulder blades together. Hold that squeeze as maximally as possible for 7-10 seconds, then relax. You should feel this in the central portion of your back between your shoulder blades out to your shoulders.

Chest

You can work your chest by grabbing both elbows with each hand with arms crossed in front of you, and try to pull each arm across your body while flexing your chest muscles. You can also activate your chest muscles by pushing your palms together in front of your chest while tensioning your chest muscles.

Biceps

You can work your biceps by holding your hands in front of your stomach, elbows bent. If you are working your right arm, your right palm will be facing up, and your left palm will be facing down. Push down with your left hand and pull up with your right hand with maximal strain of your biceps muscle.

Triceps

The triceps can be worked in a similar manner by holding the hands together out in front of you, but instead of trying to flex your elbow, this time you will concentrate on trying to extend your elbow while pulling back and resisting with the opposite hand.

Quadriceps

Lower body exercises can be performed as well using isometric techniques. Quadriceps activation can be done by placing your leg out in front of you (either on the floor or extended at the knee with the foot in the air) and tightening the quadriceps muscle (the muscle that travels from your hip to your knee down the front of your thigh. As with all of these isometric exercises, really concentrate on making that muscle as tight as possible and hold for 7-10 seconds. The back side of your thigh and glutes can be worked when sitting down in your chair if you bring your knee up slightly with your foot off the floor and grab the front of your leg just below your knee with both hands, fingers interlocked. Pull back with your hands while pushing your knee down and out away from your body.

You can also perform isometric squats by "sitting" at your desk without your chair and trying to hold this sitting position for as long as possible. Keep your feet just wider than shoulder width and bend hips and knees to as low as where your thighs become parallel to the floor. Time how long you can hold this position and then try to beat that time later.

Calf muscles

You can work your calf muscles by slightly pointing your foot and tightening your calf muscles while focusing on the area behind your lower leg.

Abdominals

An exercise that can be done to work your abdominals was popularized by bodybuilders such as Arnold Schwarzenegger and is known as vacuum's. This exercise is performed by sitting up straight in your chair and exhaling as much as possible. Then, hold your breath and suck in your stomach as much as possible. Try to imagine your belly-button touching your spine. Hold for 7-10 seconds, then relax. You can repeat this a few times. As you get more practice, you can work on holding this pose for longer.

STRETCHING

People with desk jobs especially are prone to develop muscle imbalances, causing pain and stiffness. One fix for this is to quit your job and find a new one. If that doesn't appeal to you, another option to decrease your pain is to identify your imbalances and work to improve them.

An easy way to understand how muscle imbalances develop is to think of a tight, short muscle opposed by a long, flexible muscle. One example is tight, strong chest muscles opposed by loose, weak upper back muscles. This is caused by a hunched over position while sitting and working on a computer for 8 hours a day. Another common example is tight hip flexors (again, from sitting) that will pull your pelvis forward and cause low back pain. Weak abs are opposed by tight hamstrings and cause protrusion of your belly.

An efficient stretching program is a crucial component to your overall health and will maximize your ability to realize gains from strength training. We recommend at least 10 minutes of stretching following your workouts. As an example, we will examine the cause and treatment for the "rounded shoulder" posture we see so often in clinic as it contributes to shoulder pain.

Has your mother reminded you to stand up straight recently? If so, you may benefit from the following process. You likely have rounding of your thoracic spine (postural thoracic kyphosis), tightness of your shoulder (subscapularis), upper shoulder blade muscles (trapezius and levator scapuli), and chest (pectoralis minor). All of these tight muscles will have to be stretched. Going back to our basic principle, every tight muscle will be opposed by weak muscles that we have to strengthen.

Thoracic mobility exercises, focusing primarily on extension will be the key to fix the rounded back. The subscapularis will be opposed by the external rotators of the shoulder (infraspinatus and teres minor), the upper shoulder blade by the lower shoulder blade (lower trapezius and rhomboids), the chest by the serratus anterior. Your doctor, a local physical therapist, and even the internet can be great resources for muscle-specific stretching and strengthening exercises using minimal equipment.

The above example will not apply to everyone, but we hope you see the importance in evaluating what hurts and using exercise to fix it. Table 5.6 contains some basic stretches that you can use to get started, in conjunction with consultation with your doctor. Hold each stretch for a minimum of 10 seconds.

Stretch	Description
Posterior shoulder stretch	Bring one arm across the front of your body at shoulder level and use the other arm to grab at the level of the elbow to pull your arm further across the front of your body and stretch the back of your shoulder.
Shoulder overhead stretch	Clasp both hands together with your arms straight and bring your hands up overhead as high and as far back as you can reach them.
Chest stretch	Similar to the overhead stretch, clasp both hands behind your back with arms straight and reach up behind your back as far as possible.

Stretch (cont'd)	Description
Single side chest stretch	With arm straight, reach out to the side and as far back as possible with your hand against a wall. Turn your body to the side opposite the arm you are stretching in order to stretch your chest muscles.
Gluteal stretch	Lying flat while flexing the hip and knee, grab the knee with one arm and the foot with the other hand and pull toward your chest while you feel the stretch in your gluteal muscles.
Hamstring stretch	Seated with feet out in front of you, lean forward trying to touch your toes with knees as straight as possible.
Achilles/Plantar fascia stretch	Seated with one foot resting on the opposite knee (legs partially crossed) grab the ball of your foot and pull your forefoot back toward your shin to stretch your Achilles. Next bring your hand up over your toes with fingers pointed back toward your heel and pull again while concentrating on stretching the bottom of your foot (plantar fascia).

Table 5.6—Example Stretches that Can Be Performed to Help Improve Muscle/Tissue Tightness

As you can hopefully see from this chapter, realizing the health benefits from exercising does not take hours every day in a gym or running until your cartilage is worn down to bone. Even small amounts of exercise can help tremendously toward achieving good health if done in the right way.

Find exercises that fit into your schedule and ones that you find interesting and fun (or at least find exercises you don't hate) so that you can stay motivated enough to do them. As you become comfortable with simple exercises, consider experimenting with more advanced exercises and routines as you can tolerate them. Remember why you are doing this – to get healthy – and hopefully this chapter can help you on that path.

6 | HARD AND HEALTHY BONES

BONE AND OTHER SOFT TISSUE DISORDERS

Bone disease (specifically disorders causing decreased bone density) is something that affects an estimated 50 million Americans every year in profound ways. Every year, 2 million Americans sustain fractures related to poor bone quality. These fractures most often occur as a result of an underlying disease process that can weaken the entire skeleton and can commonly be accompanied by morbid conditions that can lead to decreased function and even to an increased risk of death when these fractures occur.

While some weakening of bone throughout a lifetime is inevitable, there is much that can be done to improve bone health through diet, supplementation, exercise, and in some cases prescription medication. We have written this chapter to serve as a guide to help get you on a path to better bone health by making good lifestyle choices, and by having the right discussions with your doctor to keep your bones as healthy as they can be.

HOW DO I KNOW IF THE INFORMATION
IN THIS CHAPTER IS PERTINENT TO ME?

First, we want to tell you that even if this information is not immediately pertinent to you and your health, there is most likely someone in your life that you know and care about for whom this chapter is vitally important. The knowledge that you gain here may allow you to help them get on a course to prevent serious problems in the future they did not even know they were at risk of. Additionally, if you plan on living long enough, no matter who you are this information will become pertinent so we encourage you to read on.

Some of the risk factors of developing brittle bones (osteoporosis) and, therefore, fractures related to the disease (fragility fractures), include female gender, increasing age, low calcium and vitamin D levels, long-term steroid use, family history of brittle bones, sedentary lifestyle, and tobacco use. Other factors, such as some medical conditions and the use of certain medications exist as risk factors also. Osteoporosis causes the density of bones to become decreased, which makes them more susceptible to breaking even from minor trauma. In many cases, people do not even become aware of the presence of this problem until after they have developed one of these fragility fractures. Because these fractures can lead to decreased function and increased mortality, it is important to recognize risk factors and work to increase bone density to the degree possible before these fractures occur.

Low energy fractures of the spine, hip, and wrist are common in people with osteoporosis. In fact, when these fractures occur in an elderly person after a ground level fall they should be cause enough to at least prompt a visit to a doctor to discuss osteoporosis and consider further testing. Diagnosis of osteoporosis is made by bone densitometry testing (DEXA scan). Laboratory work such as vitamin D and calcium levels will often be checked as well.

HOW CAN I HELP PREVENT/DELAY OSTEOPOROSIS?

As you have just read, one of the risk factors for osteoporosis is advancing age. For those reading this book, preventing this risk factor entirely will likely not be desirable. Therefore, the goal is to focus on some of the other *modifiable* risk factors that you can control, to ultimately decrease your risk of developing fragility fractures. Diagnostic assessment should be sought by individuals who have one or several of the above risk factors.

Women over the age of 65 and men over the age of 70 should get a DEXA scan approximately every 3-5 years as long as their bone density measurements are normal, and every 1-2 years when abnormal testing results occur.

Postmenopausal woman under the age of 65 and any adult with height loss should also undergo DEXA scanning. The occurrence of a low energy fracture in an adult may be enough to prompt a DEXA scan and treatment. Adults with a history of long-term steroid use should also seek a doctor's opinion regarding bone density testing.

In addition to regular monitoring of bone density for those at risk of osteoporosis, there are several lifestyle choices you can make to help keep your bones hard and healthy. Regular resistance exercises (see Chapter 5) can help to strengthen bones and can further reduce the risk of falls and fragility fractures by increasing muscle tone, endurance, and agility. Resistance training can be performed by people of all ages, body types, and strength. It is important to start with a program that is appropriate for your current fitness level, and gradually increase the intensity as you get stronger.

Adequate calcium and vitamin D intake is essential in combating osteoporosis as you age. As mentioned above, speaking with your doctor and measuring calcium and vitamin D levels is important as you age and develop risk factors for brittle bones. Recommendations by the National Osteoporosis Foundation includes calcium intake of 1200 mg/day for women over 50 and men over 70, and 1000 mg/day for men age 50-70. Vitamin D intake is recommended to be 800-1000 IU/day for all individuals age 50 and older.[50] For those who do not routinely reach these levels in their regular diet (which is common), a dietary supplement of calcium and vitamin D is recommended. Too much calcium or vitamin D (as it is with too much of anything) can cause problems to develop. Therefore, if unsure as to whether or not a calcium and vitamin D supplementation is appropriate for you, we recommend consultation with your physician.

As if you didn't already know about enough of the detriments of smoking, yet another reason to quit all nicotine use is that it can increase your risk of osteoporosis and fragility fracture. Most people are well aware of lung cancer and other cancers associated with smoking, but far fewer people are aware of the detrimental effects of nicotine on bone health. If not for many other reasons, nicotine use should be discontinued to promote hard and healthy bones.

WHAT HAPPENS IF I'M DIAGNOSED WITH OSTEOPOROSIS?

When a fragility fracture has occurred and/or osteoporosis has been diagnosed by DEXA scan, pharmacologic treatment is often indicated.

Your doctor will review your individual situation and will most likely prescribe medication. There are several different medications that can be used to prevent or even reverse some of the bone density loss that occurs with the disease. Which medication is best for you will be determined by your doctor. The length of time you will need to be on these medications is also variable according to your specific situation. As stated above, calcium and vitamin D supplementation will often be a part of the treatment of osteoporosis as well.

OSTEOPOROSIS AND METABOLIC SYNDROME

As mentioned earlier in this book, metabolic syndrome can have detrimental effects on the body including development of heart disease, diabetes, and stroke. Metabolic syndrome is characterized by having three or more of the following traits: 1) abdominal obesity (large waist circumference of 35 inches for women, 40 for men), 2) high blood pressure, 3) dyslipidemia (high triglyceride and low HDL), and 4) elevated blood sugar. Recent research has attempted to determine whether or not there is a relationship between metabolic syndrome and osteoporosis. Because osteoporosis is such a widespread and devastating disease, an understanding of the relationship between metabolic syndrome and osteoporosis could help to prevent or reverse osteoporosis for some people.

Obesity and increased body mass index (BMI) have long been thought to be protective against osteoporosis and osteoporotic fractures.[51] Recent evidence, however, has challenged this belief. Recent animal studies have shown detrimental effects on bone mineral density in cases where diet-induced metabolic syndrome has been introduced.[52,53] Moreover, when specific components of the metabolic syndrome were created in animal models (such as hyperglycemia, hypertension, etc.), numerus detrimental effects on bone were found such as decreased bone mineral density, decreased bone strength, etc.[54-57] These findings have in large part been consistent in the human literature. While some human studies have in fact suggested a protective effect on bone density from increased body mass as mentioned above, when researchers have controlled for the mechanical effect on bones from increased BMI they have shown a detrimental effect on bone density from obesity.[58] Additionally, when subgroup analyses have been performed, several studies have shown detrimental effects on bone mineral density in men associated with metabolic syndrome, especially with larger waist sizes.[59-63] This means that for unknown reasons, metabolic syndrome particularly affects men in a more negative way in terms of bone mineral density than it does women. Furthermore, as BMI increases to varying levels of obesity, the benefit to bone density does not increase and eventually begins to be associated with decreasing bone mineral density in both men and women.[64] Still, in other studies that have shown a positive effect on bone mineral density with metabolic syndrome, there has been no apparent benefit in fracture reduction in these same groups.[65]

While the association between metabolic syndrome and osteoporosis is a complex one, it is clear that the negative effects of metabolic syndrome far outweigh any potential protective benefit to bones. Resistance exercises can provide the benefit of mechanical loading to bones, without the numerus health problems that are accompanied with increasing BMI. Osteoporosis is a complex disease that can be significantly affected by lifestyle choices. This is yet another area of life where proper diet and exercise can go a long way.

SOFT TISSUE DISORDERS[66]

Other musculoskeletal changes are seen in greater frequency in association with poor diet and metabolic abnormalities. While these conditions are seen in non-diabetics as well, an increased incidence of these pathologies are seen in people with diabetes. Disorders such as frozen shoulder, carpal tunnel syndrome, and trigger finger are seen in greater frequency in diabetics. Neuropathy (abnormal nerve function that is also often painful) can result in foot ulcers that may have prolonged healing times or even lead to amputation. Charcot arthropathy (rapid and severe destruction of joints) is a condition that arises more frequently in diabetics and can result in loss of function, need for surgery, and in some cases loss of limb. These conditions can at times be prevented by recognizing and correcting problems with glucose metabolism prior to the onset of these ailments.

Although often a byproduct of gaining maturity (a nice way of saying getting older), many of these conditions can be prevented, reversed, or at least controlled in part or completely with the proper diet and exercise. What is "proper" for you will depend on your current health status, exercise experience, etc. Please discuss these issues with your physician and bone up on your health.

7 | KETOGENIC AND
INTELLIGENT CARB RECIPES

As discussed in detail in Chapter 4, your meals will mostly consist of a combination of protein from meat and of carbohydrates from sources such as vegetables and beans that are rich sources of fiber and vitamins. You can have a relatively short shopping list and a few things that you cook, but by mixing and matching from the various foods on that list and using different sauces/spices you can have a lot of variety in what you eat. Although fully compliant Intelligent Carb meals can be made with little thought or effort in a short amount of time as discussed previously, recipes can be found here and online (www.intelligentcarb.com/recipes).

With all recipes keep in mind that if you see an ingredient that you don't like, try the recipe without it, or with another low carb substitute. These recipes are simply a guide to help you find some good tasting meals but feel free to tailor them to your specific tastes. If there is a low carb ingredient that you don't see that you want to add, feel free to do that as well. Enjoy!

SAMPLE INTELLIGENT CARB MEALS
AND COMPONENT PARTS

MIXED VEGETABLES

Pan fry, grill, bake, steam, etc., however you like them. Cook with MCT oil or butter. Add some seasoning such as Montreal Steak Seasoning or a chili sauce.

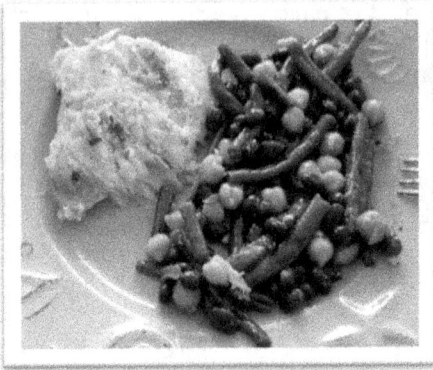

Baked chicken with green bean/ garbanzo bean/black bean salad.

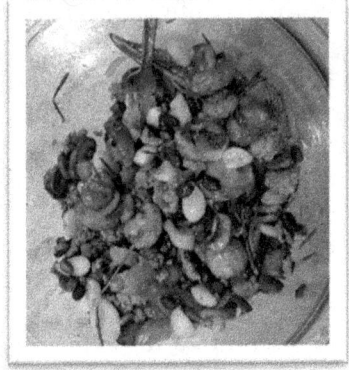

ground turkey with shallots/ onions/black beans/mushrooms

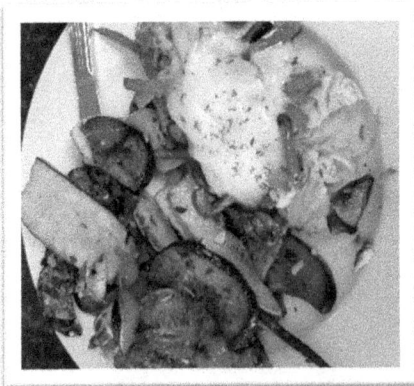

baked chicken and cheese with red peppers/zucchini/eggplant/ yellow squash

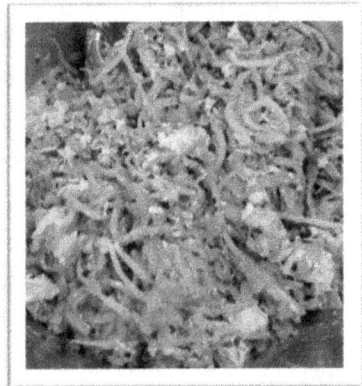

"Pad Thai" with chicken/carrots/ zucchini/bean sprouts

CAULIFLOWER MASHED POTATOES

Take cauliflower and cut into small pieces (or buy riced cauliflower), then boil or steam until soft. Place in a blender or food processor with butter, salt, and pepper. Cream cheese can be added as well.

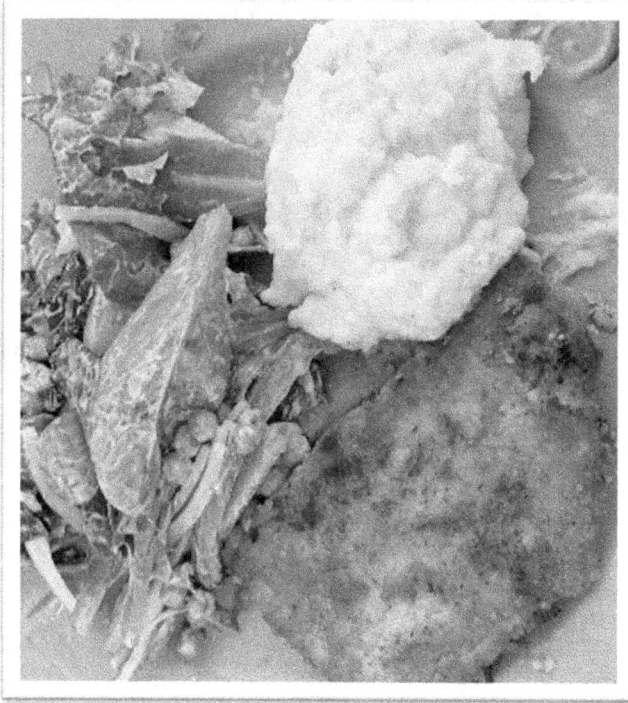

Pork crusted with almond flour,
mixed green salad with mayo
dressing, and mashed cauliflower

TACO MEAT

Ground beef and refried beans. Place in a pan and sprinkle with taco seasoning. Heat in pan.

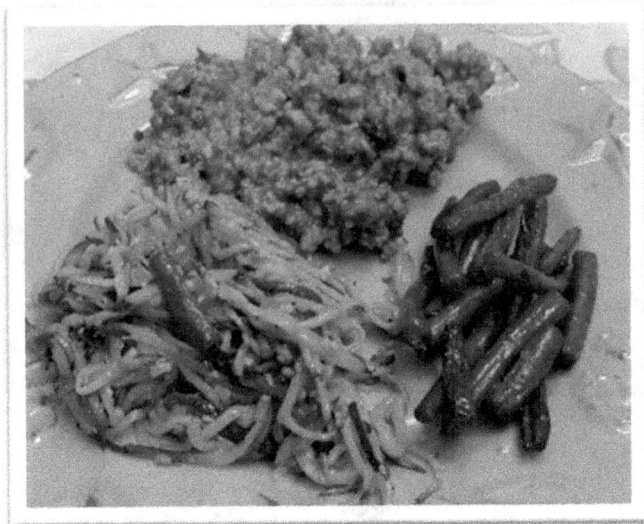

*Taco meat with zucchini noodles
sautéed in butter with green beans*

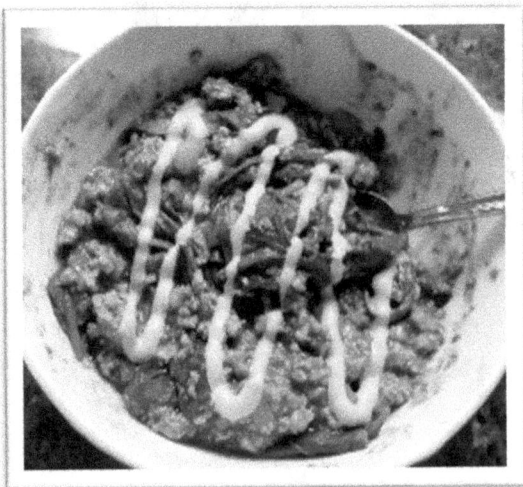

*Taco meat with spinach
and sriracha mayo*

STEAK

Cook it in a pan on high heat to brown the outside. Next, place it in an oven at 350 degrees and check every 5 minutes until cooked to desired center heat.

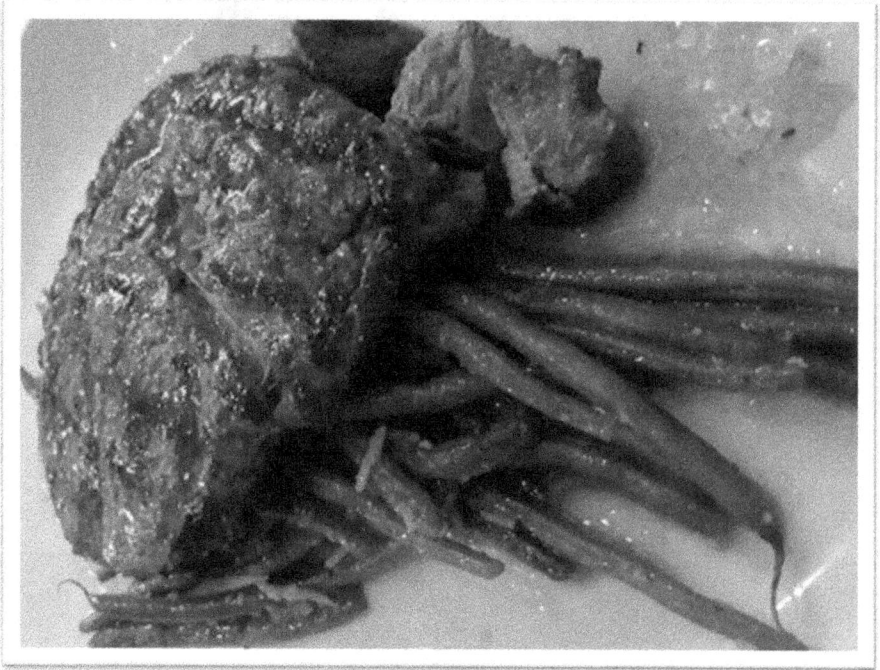

Ribeye steak with green beans

SALADS

Add any of the approved ingredients from Table 4.1 as desired. Mayonnaise or balsamic vinaigrette can be used for dressing. Many low carb dressings are available commercially as well. Black beans, hard boiled eggs, chicken, etc., all make great additions to a salad.

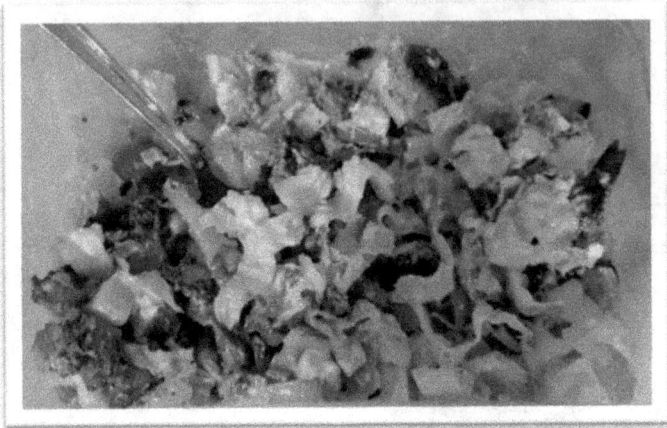

Ground beef/red pepper/yellow pepper salad

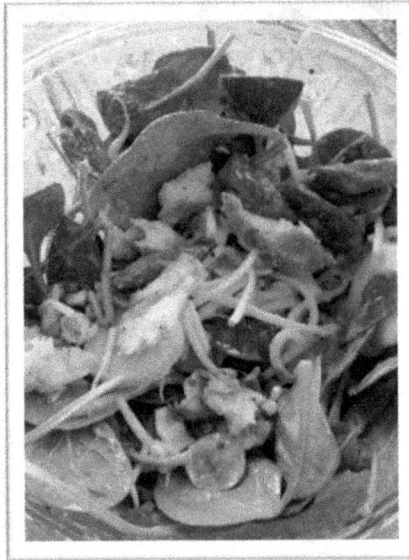

Fish/spinach/bean sprouts salad

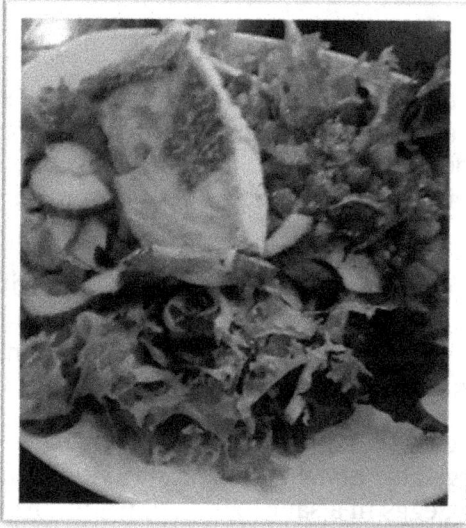

Fish/cucumber/salsa/salad

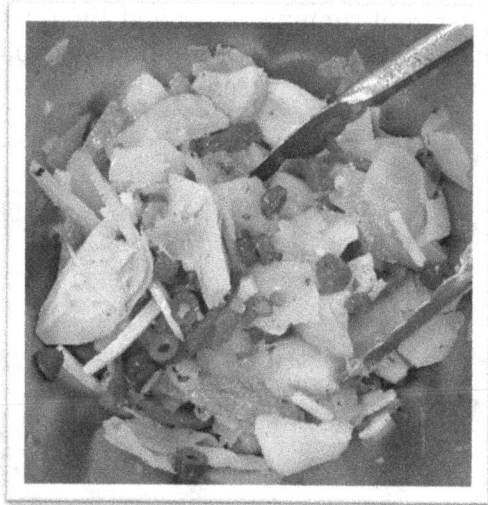

*artichoke/cabbage/olive/
salami/roasted red pepper/
capers antipasto*

ROASTED KALE

Place kale on a baking sheet, drizzle with olive oil and sprinkle with salt. Cook at 350 degrees for 20 minutes. Remove from the oven and add some walnuts, toss, and serve.

EGGS

Okay, everybody knows how to make an egg, right? Well, we hope so but we put this in not to give a "recipe," but to stress the points that we believe eggs are such a great food source that can help you on your journey to get healthy and they are so convenient to have around as a healthy protein source.

Take a desired amount of whole eggs or one whole egg and mix it with egg whites (or use cartons of pre-prepared egg-whites). Whisk, then scramble in a pan to desired consistency. Eggs can also be cooked in a microwave for approximately 45 seconds for one egg.

Also, try to keep some hard boiled eggs in the fridge for mornings when you're in a rush. Hard boiled eggs also make a great addition to other meals as well. Prepare by placing eggs in a saucepan with water, bring water to a boil, then simmer on low heat for 12 minutes. Place saucepan under cool running water and then remove eggs. Tip: place baking soda in the water. Depending on your stove and your ideal egg doneness, you may need to adjust the simmer time up or down.

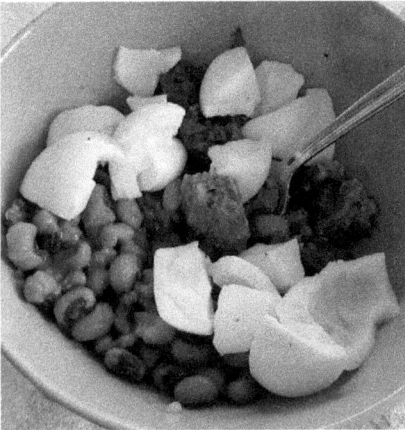

ground beef/boiled egg whites/
black eyed peas

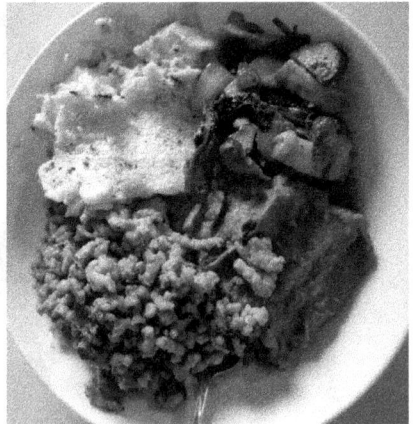

ground turkey/scrambled eggs/
refried beans/mushroom/spinach/onion

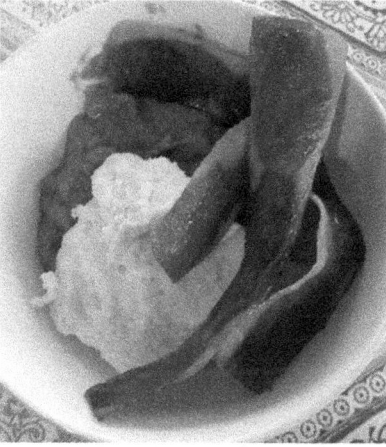

scrambled eggs/refried beans/
turkey bacon

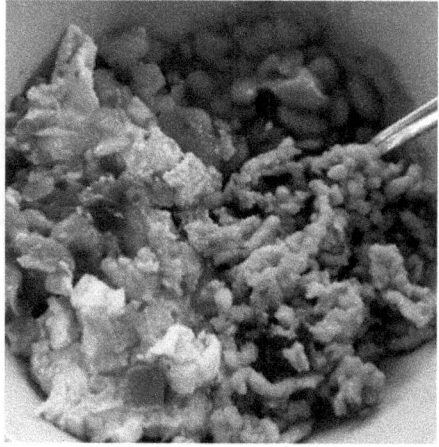

ground turkey/scrambled eggs/
grilled peppers/pinto beans

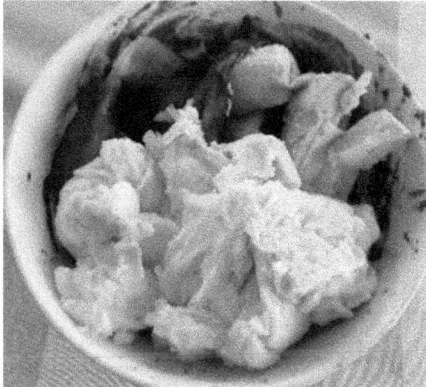

scrambled eggs/black beans/
avocado/bacon

INTELLIGENT CARB MEATBALLS

Ingredients
1 lb. ground beef
½ c almond flour
1 egg
1 T Montreal steak seasoning
½ onion, chopped (optional)
1 green chile, chopped (optional)

Preheat oven to 400 degrees. Mix ground beef, almond flour, egg and seasoning into a bowl. Add optional ingredients if desired. Line a baking dish with tinfoil and cooking spray. Form meatballs into desired shape and size and place in dish. Bake uncovered for 20-25 minutes.

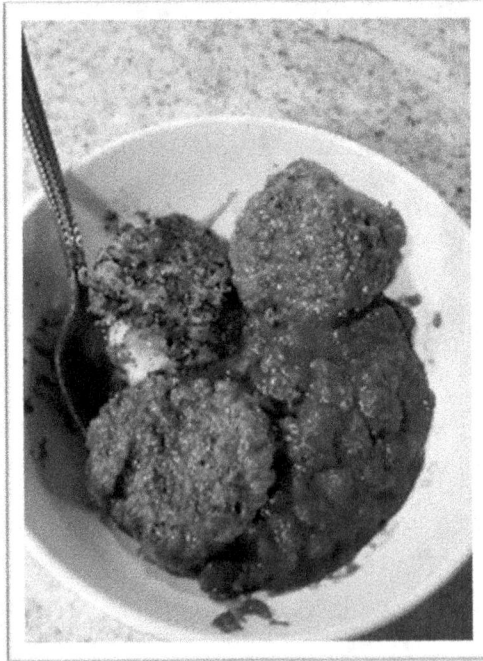

Intelligent Carb Meatballs/
broccoli/black beans

ANYTIME CHICKEN

Ingredients
1 lb. chicken breast
1 c olive oil
1 T garlic salt
2 t basil
1 T paprika
3 T Montreal steak seasoning
2 lemons

Mix (whisk) olive oil, garlic salt, basil, paprika, and Montreal steak seasoning. Drizzle some of this mixture on a 9" x 13" glass pan and then place chicken in pan and coat both sides with the olive oil mixture. Next squeeze lemon juice on top. Cook chicken for 15 min at 450 degrees. Flip chicken over and baste, squeezing on more lemon juice. Cook 10 min, then flip, baste and squeeze additional lemon juice. Cook 15 min more.

This recipe can also be done with a crockpot or Instapot. Place chicken in a crockpot. Take olive oil mixture and pour on top of chicken. Squeeze on lemon juice. Set crockpot on low for 8 hours, or high for 6 hours. When done remove chicken and shred with two forks. Serve or save for later (this chicken is great even cold or heated up as leftovers).

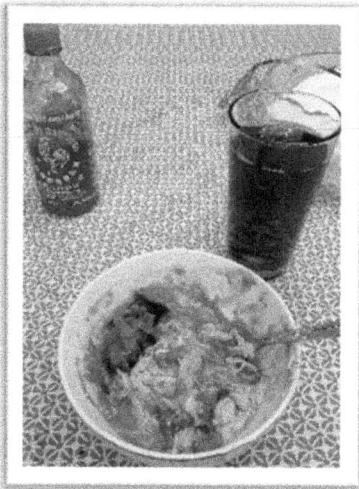

*Chicken/spinach/
refried beans/sriracha*

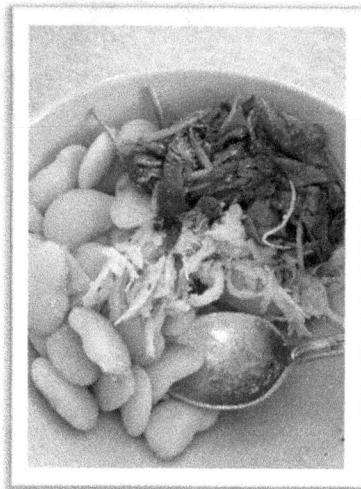

Chicken/butter beans/spinach

BUFFALO CHICKEN DIP

Ingredients
½ to 1 lb. shredded chicken (I have also substituted with ground turkey here from time to time)
5 T hot sauce (Franks Red Hot Buffalo) or more to taste
one 8 oz pkg cream cheese
¼ c low carb ranch dressing (or mayonnaise, or blue cheese dressing)
2 c mozzarella or cheddar cheese, shredded

Preheat oven to 350 degrees. Heat cream cheese until soft in a saucepan or covered in the microwave, add hot sauce, and stir until fully combined. Add low carb ranch dressing and continue to stir. Color should be orange, if too light may need to add more hot sauce. Mix with chicken. Mix in about half of the cheese. Spread mixture in a baking dish and sprinkle with the remainder of the cheese. Place in the oven for 15 minutes, or until cheese on top has melted.

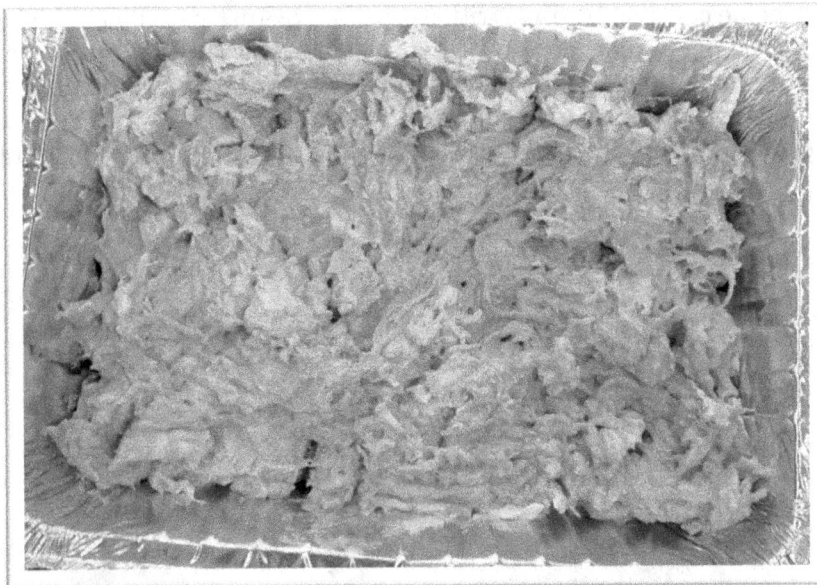

Buffalo chicken dip

OVEN BAKED BEANS

Ingredients
3 c dry beans (kidney, black, pinto)
2 t chili powder
1 t dry mustard
6 T dry white wine
1 ½ t salt

Opt. ingredients
2 c chopped onion
1 c diced green peppers
1 c chopped turkey, ham, or bacon, etc.

Remove three cups of raw beans of your choice (kidney, black, pinto, etc.) from the bag. Sift and sort (remove any dirt or broken beans). Rinse and soak for several hours or overnight if possible. Place beans in a large pot and cover with water. Cook on a stovetop for 90 minutes or more until beans are done to desired consistency. Drain.

Sauté the onion, peppers, and meat in butter. Add the chili powder and dry mustard. Remove from heat and add this mixture to the cooked beans and remaining ingredients. Pour all into a large buttered casserole dish. Cover and bake at 350 degrees for 40 minutes.

CREAMY KALE

Ingredients
5 T butter
2 T almond flour
½ t cinnamon
¼ t pepper
¼ t salt

1 c chicken stock
1 ½ c heavy cream
3 bags kale (8 oz each)
1 c parmesan cheese (optional)
1 onion (optional)

In a saucepan, heat butter. Add almond flour and cook for 3-4 minutes, continuously stirring. Add cinnamon, salt, and pepper. Add chicken stock and cream. Continue to stir until thickened. Add kale to sauce and stir. If onions are being used, add cooked onions at this point. Stir in parmesan cheese.

BLACK-EYED PEAS

Ingredients

1 lb. dry black-eyed peas
½ lb. meat of your choice
   (pork, bacon, ham, etc.),
   bite-sized pieces
1 onion, finely chopped
1 celery stick, chopped
1 bell pepper, chopped

½ t cayenne pepper
1 t salt
¼ t pepper
1 t garlic powder
3 c chicken broth (optional)
Olive oil (if baking)

Rinse and soak beans overnight. Simmer in water or chicken broth in a saucepan for 90 minutes.

Preheat oven to 350 degrees. Coat a casserole dish with olive oil, then add onion, celery, and bell pepper. Drain water from beans and layer beans on top. Add spices and meat. Mix and gently mash beans. Cover with foil and bake for 40 minutes. Remove from oven, stir, and serve.

Stove-top: rinse and soak beans overnight. Add beans to a saucepan with chicken broth. Simmer for 45 minutes. Add onion, celery, bell pepper, and meat. Continue to simmer for another 45 minutes stirring occasionally. Then add spices. Mix and gently mash beans. Serve.

Slow-cooker: rinse and soak beans overnight. Add black-eyed peas and 3 cups of chicken broth, meat, onion, celery, bell pepper, and spices. Cover and cook on low for approximately 8-10 hours.

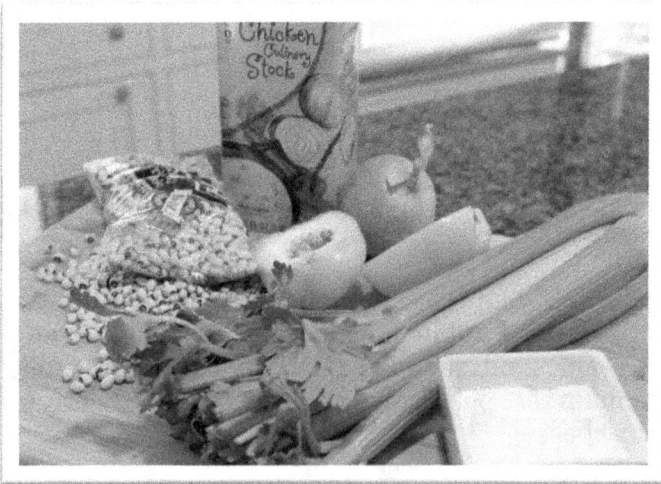

Black-eyed peas

MAKE AHEAD BREAKFAST SCRAMBLE

Ingredients
1 dozen eggs
¼ c heavy whipping cream
1 t sea salt
½ t pepper
2 T butter
½ lb. fully cooked turkey sausage, crumbled
1 can black beans, drained
2c shredded Mexican blend cheese
1 bunch green onions, chopped
6 small storage containers

Whisk together eggs, cream, salt, and pepper in a large bowl. Then, heat butter in a large nonstick skillet. As soon as butter is melted add egg mixture. When eggs are cooked to your liking, add sausage, beans and 1 cup of cheese and mix well until sausage is warmed and cheese is melted.

Transfer 1 cup of the egg mixture to storage containers (makes six 1-cup portions). Top with remaining cheese and green onions divided evenly among 6 portions. Let cool for 10 minutes, then put the lids on the storage containers. Store in refrigerator. Use within 7 days.

To reheat, remove lid and cover with damp paper towel. Microwave for 1-½ minutes, stir and enjoy.

BACON BRUSSELS

Ingredients
2 lbs. Brussels sprouts, cored and cut in half
¼ c butter
2/3 c pine nuts
½ lb. bacon
3 green onions, minced
Salt and pepper, to taste (about ½ - 1 teaspoon each)

Cook bacon in a pan on the stove, cut or crumble, then set aside. In that pan, melt the butter, add the pine nuts, and cook until pine nuts are toasted (brown). Then add the Brussels sprouts, onions, and seasoning. As the Brussels sprouts are nearly cooked, add in the bacon.

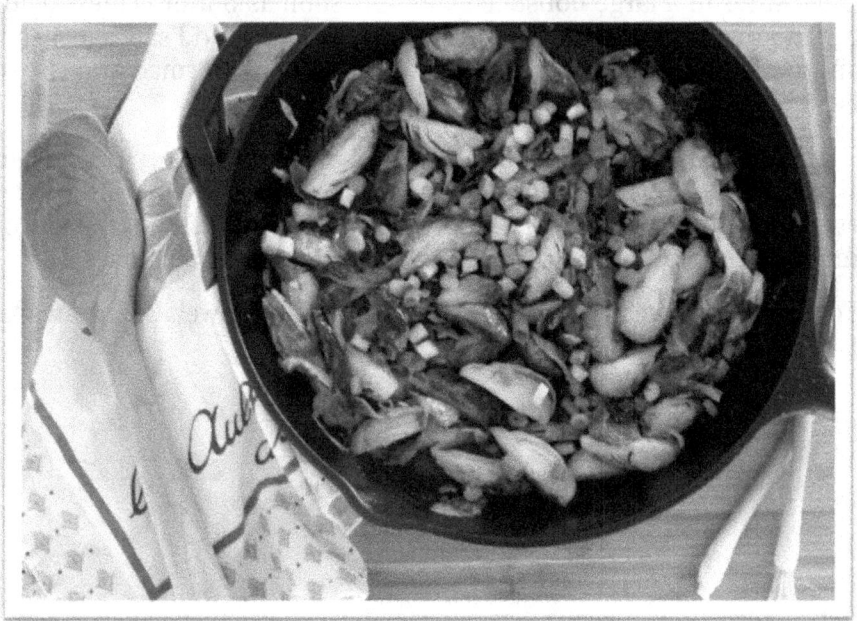

Bacon Brussels

CAULIFLOWER BREAD

Ingredients
1 head cauliflower, chopped with stems removed
½ c parmesan cheese, shredded
1 egg
1 t garlic herb seasoning (or similar seasoning of your preference)

Preheat oven to 450 degrees. Place cauliflower in a food processor and grind to pieces smaller than a grain of rice. Cook until soft and then dry cauliflower (15 minutes in the microwave, stirring once every 3 minutes while cooking will accomplish this). Next, add the egg, parmesan cheese, and seasoning. Mix until the result is a "doughy" smooth paste.

Place onto a large baking sheet with parchment paper in desired size (4 equal parts for bread, all in one ½-inch thick piece for pizza crust, etc.). Bake until golden brown (about 15 minutes).

Use your "bread" to make your desired meal. Place a burger patty and cheese between two slices and keep in the oven for another 10 minutes to make patty melt. Place butter in a pan and cook on the stove while placing turkey and cheese in between two slices to make a turkey melt (flip carefully). Add pizza sauce, cheese, and any other toppings of your choice to make pizza. Get creative.

Makes 4 pieces of bread/mini pizza crust/breadsticks, etc.

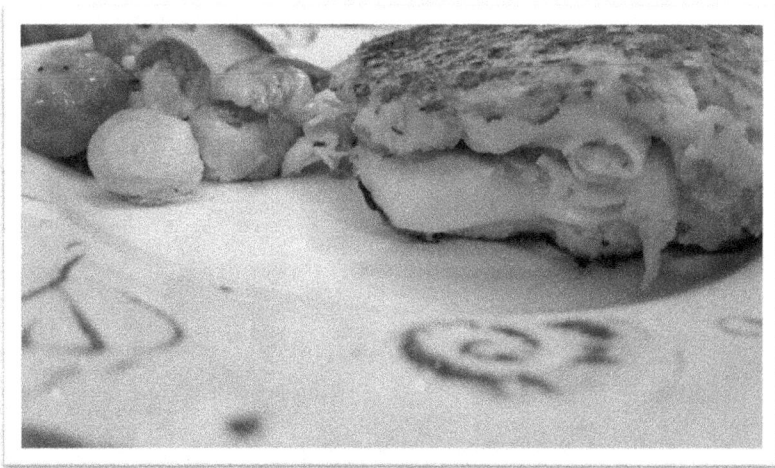

Cauliflower turkey melt with Brussels sprouts (see previous page)

BELL PEPPER NACHO MINI BOWLS

Ingredients

1 lb. ground beef

1 t chili powder

¼ t salt

¾ c salsa (low sugar, 1 gram or less per serving)

1 c Mexican cheese blend

3 bell peppers (red, yellow, orange)

1 avocado, diced (optional)

3 green onions, diced (optional)

sour cream (optional)

1 t cumin

½ t black pepper

Preheat oven to 375 degrees. Slice bell peppers in half lengthwise and remove seeds, core, and membranes. Set peppers aside.

In a nonstick pan, cook ground beef until cooked through and no longer pink, breaking it up as it cooks. Drain off any fat. Combine cooked beef with spices and salsa. Evenly distribute the beef mixture into the bell pepper halves and top with cheese.

Bake on a lined baking sheet (either parchment or foil) for 10 minutes or until cheese is melted and peppers are hot. Serve with diced avocado, sour cream, and/or diced green onions.

Note: If you prefer softer bell pepper, then add ¼ cup of water to bottom of a casserole dish, add filled peppers, cover tightly with foil and bake for 15 minutes.

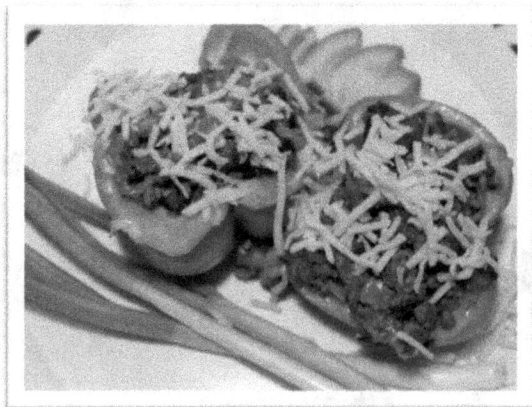

Bell Pepper Nacho Mini Bowls

CHICKEN AVOCADO CUPS

Ingredients
4 avocados, halved and pitted
4 cans canned chicken (6 oz each, drained)
1 t chili powder
1 T cilantro, finely chopped
½ t salt
¼ t pepper
1 lime
4 oz soft cream cheese (or mayonnaise)
½ c mozzarella cheese (optional)
4 slices bacon, chopped (optional)
sriracha mayo, to taste (optional)

Combine chicken, chili powder, salt, pepper, cilantro, bacon (if desired), and cream cheese into a bowl, and mix together. Place this mixture into the avocado halves and sprinkle with lime juice and cheese. Serve cold or place in a baking dish and bake at 400 degrees for 10 minutes.

Tip: another great keto snack is a variation on this. Take half an avocado and sprinkle with 1 tablespoon of MCT oil and crushed macadamia nuts and enjoy.

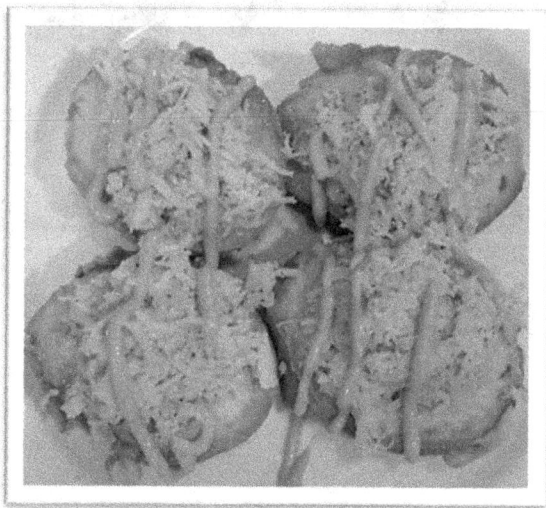

Chicken avocado cups with sriracha mayo

SOUTHWEST LIME SALMON

Ingredients
2 limes for zest/juice
2 T chili powder
½ t salt
4 salmon fillets
2 T olive oil

Zest lime; squeeze limes for juice. Combine zest, juice, chili powder, and salt; reserve 1 tablespoon mixture. Preheat large nonstick sauté pan on medium. Brush salmon with chili mixture. Place oil in pan, then add salmon; cook 3 minutes on each side and until 145 degrees and separates easily. Using a clean brush, coat top of salmon with reserved chili mixture and serve.

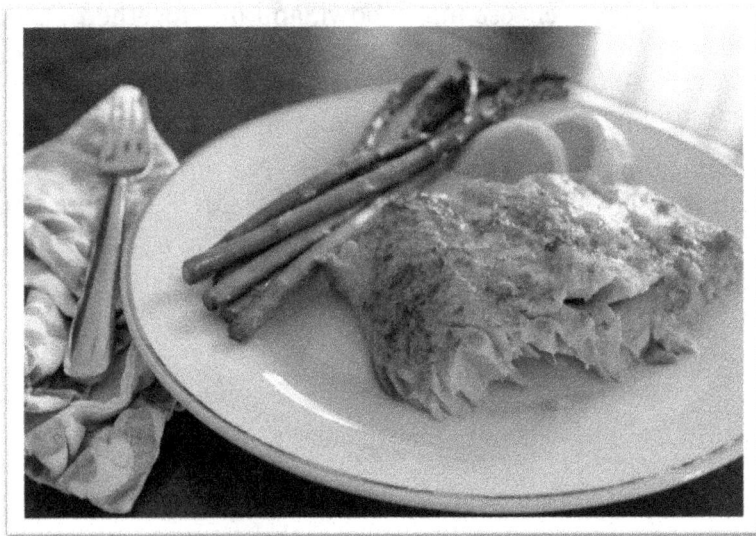

Salmon and asparagus

MEATZA

Ingredients
1 lb. your choice of meat (ground beef, ground turkey,
     finely shredded or ground chicken)
1 egg
1 c provolone
1 c mozzarella cheese (or other preferred cheese such as parmesan)
½ c low carb pizza sauce
10 slices pepperoni (or other desired topping)
½ t or more based on your preference:

garlic salt	caraway seeds
oregano	black pepper
red pepper flakes	thyme

Preheat oven to 400 degrees. Mix meat, egg, and spices together.
Spread meat out in a thin layer on a baking dish in desired shape. Cook
for about 10 minutes until meat appears cooked throughout. Remove
from oven and top with cheese, sauce, pepperoni, and more cheese.
Place back into the oven to melt cheese (about 3 minutes).

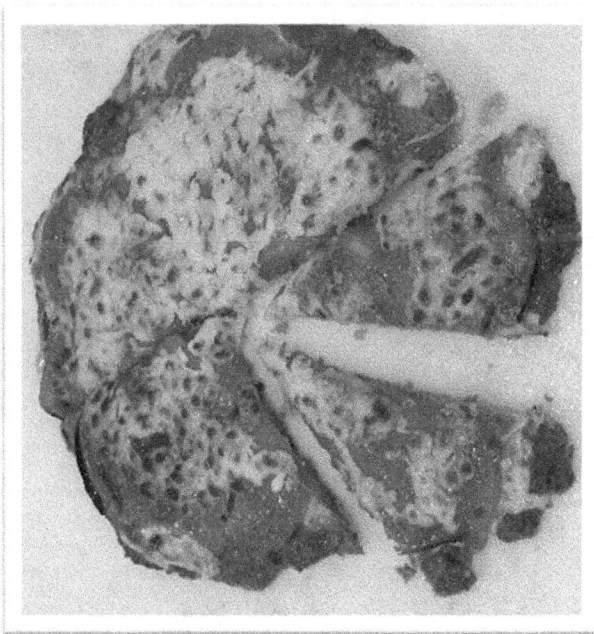

Pepperoni meatza

KETO PIZZA

Ingredients
2/3 c coconut flour
1 t baking powder
Italian seasoning (or other spices to taste)
2+1 eggs
1 ½ c shredded mozzarella (or parmesan) cheese

Preheat oven to 425 degrees. Beat 2 eggs and mix in spices, baking powder, coconut flour, and cheese. Mix dough thoroughly. In order to make dough more workable at this stage, it may help to mix in another egg followed by two tablespoons of water.

Spread dough over greased parchment paper. Bake for 15 minutes, checking periodically for bubbles in the crust (pop with a fork if present). Remove and let sit 5 min, then flip. Place low carb toppings of your choice (if using tomato sauce use low carb sauce, 3-4 g or less), cheese, meat, vegetables, etc. Place back into the oven and cook approximately 10 min longer.

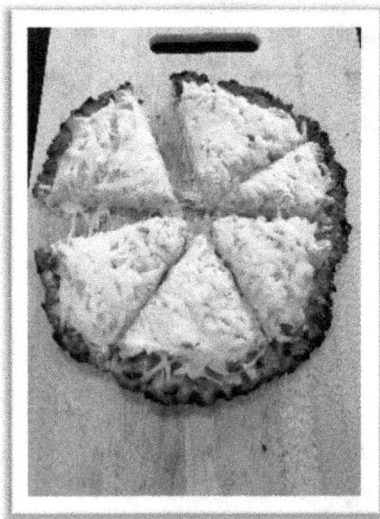

Buffalo chicken low-carb pizza

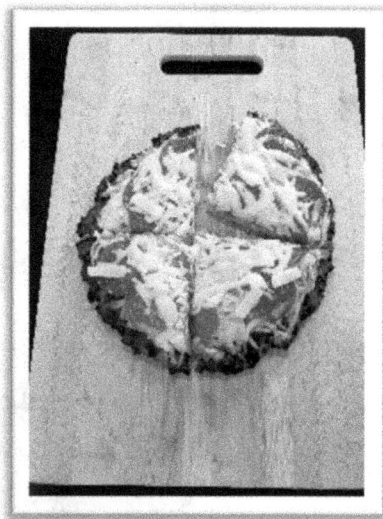

Pepperoni and onion low-carb pizza

TUNA CEVICHE

Ingredients
1 lb. sushi grade tuna, raw or cooked
½ c onion, finely chopped
½ c cilantro, chopped
½ c tomato, finely chopped
¼ c zucchini, raw, shredded
1 avocado, diced
¼ c lime juice
¼ c lemon juice
½ t salt
¼ t pepper

Soak the tuna (or other fish if desired) in the lime juice, lemon juice, salt, and pepper. Soak for at least 20-30 minutes (cook at this point if desired), then add onion, cilantro, tomatoes, and zucchini and mix all together. Chill until ready to serve. Add avocado just before serving.

CHICKEN AND PEPPERS

Ingredients
10 chicken breast strips, cut into cubes
1 red pepper, cubed
5 habanero peppers, sliced
1 onion, sliced
1 avocado, cut in half
1 t salt

Cook chicken in MCT oil in a pan on stovetop and sprinkle with salt. In a separate pan cook red pepper, habanero peppers, and onion in MCT oil. Combine chicken and vegetables when nearly done. In the empty pan place avocado halves and heat briefly.

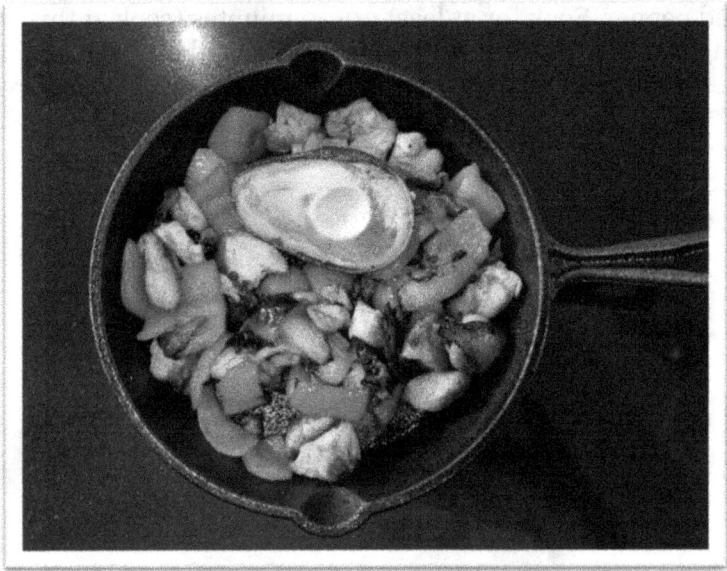

Chicken, peppers, onion, and avocado

HAMBURGER BUN

Ingredients
3 T almond flour
½ t baking powder
1 ½ t MCT oil
1 egg

In a microwave-safe bowl, mix baking powder and almond flour. Add oil and egg and mix completely. Microwave for approximately 90 seconds. Remove from microwave and dump the bun out of the bowl. Slice longways through the middle.

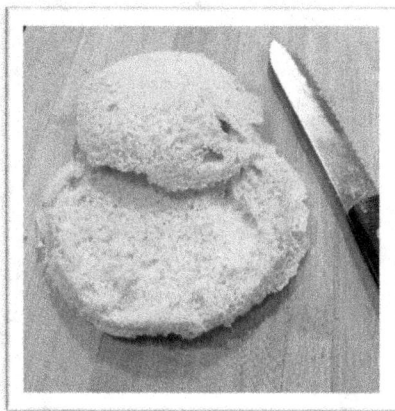

Keto bun

GREEN CURRY CHICKEN

Ingredients
Your favorite sautéed vegetables (you can also add raw spinach)
Diced and cooked meat of choice (chicken, beef, pork, shrimp)
2 jars Thai Kitchen curry paste
2 cans Thai Kitchen lite coconut milk
2 tsp Thai chili sauce

Mix all ingredients until blended. Bring to a boil. Cover and simmer on low for 10 minutes or until ready to serve.

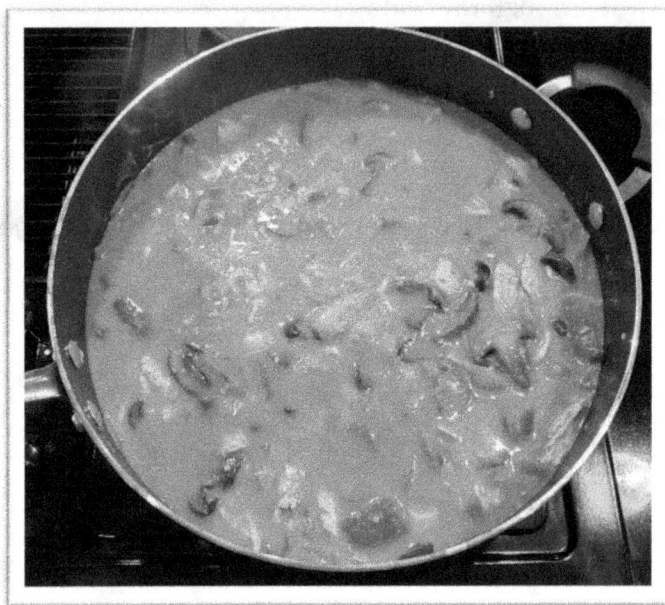

Green curry chicken

8 | CONCLUSION

Hopefully by this point you have begun to implement some of the techniques described in this book to put yourself on a pathway to better overall health. We cannot stress enough the importance of dedication as a core component to getting there, regardless of the eating plan or exercise routine.

Remind yourself often and with confidence why you are doing this – and that you will do this. Write down your goals and put them in a place where you can see them constantly. If pictures motivate you, put them in places where you can see them.

Don't get discouraged when you don't see instantaneous results – this is a marathon, not a sprint. Be most interested in long-term results including fat loss and muscle gain, not just short-term weight loss.

Measure your real success in terms of inches lost at the waist rather than pounds lost. Measure success in terms of bloodwork including lowered blood sugar, lower cholesterol, etc. And finally, measure your success by the ability to perform physical activities that you couldn't do when you first made the decision to get healthy. Good luck.

REFERENCES

[1] Stern L, Iqbal N, Seshadri P, et al. The effects of low-carbohydrate versus conventional weight loss diets in severely obese adults: one-year follow-up of a randomized trial. *Annals of Internal Medicine.* May 2004;140(10): 778-86.

[2] Paoli A, Rubini A, Volek JS, Grimaldi KA. Beyond weight loss: a review of the therapeutic uses of very-low-carbohydrate (ketogenic) diets. *European Journal of Clinical Nutrition.* Aug 2013;67(8):789-96.

[3] Hession M, Rolland C, Kulkarni U, et al. Systematic review of randomized controlled trials of low-carbohydrate vs. low-fat/low-calorie diets in the management of obesity and its comorbidities. *Obesity Reviews.* Jan 2009;10(1):36-50.

[4] Bueno NB, de Melo IS, de Oliveira SL da Rocha Ataide T. Very-low-carbohydrate ketogenic diet v. low-fat diet for long-term weight loss: a meta-analysis of randomized controlled trials. *British Journal of Nutrition.* Oct 2013;110(7):1178-87.

[5] Addison, et al. Intermuscular Fat: A Review of the Consequences and Causes. International Journal of Endocrinology. Volume 2014

[6] Goodpaster BH, Thaete FL, Kelley DE. Thigh adipose tissue distribution is associated with insulin resistance in obesity and in type 2 diabetes mellitus. American Journal of Clinical Nutrition, vol. 71, no. 4, pp. 885–892, 2000

[7] Beasley LE, Koster A, Newman AB, et al. Inflammation and race and gender differences in computerized tomography-measured adipose depots. Obesity, vol. 17, no. 5, pp. 1062–1069, 2009.

[8] Hairi NN, Cumming RG, Naganathan V, et al. Loss of muscle strength, mass (sarcopenia), and quality (specific force) and its relationship with functional limitation and physical disability: the concord health and ageing in men project. Journal of the American Geriatrics Society, vol. 58, no. 11, pp. 2055–2062, 2010.

9 Goodpaster BH, Carlson CL, Visser M, et al. Attenuation of skeletal muscle and strength in the elderly: the health ABC study. Journal of Applied Physiology, vol. 90, no. 6, pp. 2157–2165, 2001.

10 Visser M, Kritchevsky SB, Goodpaster BH, et al. Leg muscle mass and composition in relation to lower extremity performance in men and women aged 70 to 79: the Health, Aging and Body Composition Study. Journal of the American Geriatrics Society, vol. 50, no. 5, pp. 897–904, 2002.

11 Lang TJ, Cauley AF, Tylavsky, Bauer D, Cummings S, Harris TB. Computed tomographic measurements of thigh muscle cross-sectional area and attenuation coefficient predict hip fracture: the health, aging, and body composition study. Journal of Bone and Mineral Research, vol. 25, no. 3, pp. 513–519, 2010.

12 Ryan AS, Ortmeyer HK, Sorkin JD. Exercise with calorie restriction improves insulin sensitivity and glycogen synthase activity in obese postmenopausal women with impaired glucose tolerance. American Journal of Physiology: Endocrinology and Metabolism, vol. 302, no. 1, pp. E145–E152, 2012.

13 Manini TM, Clark BC, Nalls MA, Goodpaster BH, Ploutz-Snyder LL, Harris TB. Reduced physical activity increases intermuscular adipose tissue in healthy young adults. American Journal of Clinical Nutrition, vol. 85, no. 2, pp. 377–384, 2007.

14 D'Lima DD, Fregly BJ, Patil S, et al. Knee joint forces: prediction, measurement, and significance. Proc Inst Mech Eng H. Feb 2012;226(2):95-102.

15 Kabir M, Catalano KJ, Ananthnarayan S, Kim SP, Van Citters GW, Dea MK, Bergman RN. Molecular evidence supporting the portal theory: a causative link between visceral adiposity and hepatic insulin resistance. Am J Physiol Endocrinol Metab. 2005 Feb;288(2):E454-61. Epub 2004 Nov 2.

16 Tchernof A, Despres JP. Pathophysiology of human visceral obesity: an update. Physiol Rev. 2013 Jan;93(1):359-404. doi: 10.1152/physrev.00033.2011.

17 Anan F, Masaki T, Shimomura T, Fujiki M, Umeno Y, Eshima N, Saikawa T, Yoshimatsu H. Abdominal visceral fat accumulation is associated with hippocampus volume in non-dementia patients with type 2 diabetes mellitus. Neuroimage. 2010 Jan 1;49(1):57-62. doi: 10.1016/j.neuroimage.2009.08.021. Epub 2009 Aug 14.

[18] Feinman RD, Pogozelski WK, Astrup A, et al. Dietary carbohydrate restriction as the first approach in diabetes management: critical review and evidence base. Nutrition. 2015;31(1):1-13.

[19] Samaha FF, Iqbal N, Seshadri P, et al. A low-carbohydrate as compared with a low-fat diet in severe obesity. N Engl J Med. 2003;348(21):2074-81.

[20] Sondike SB, Copperman N, Jacobson MS. Effects of a low-carbohydrate diet on weight loss and cardiovascular risk factor in overweight adolescents. J Pediatr. 2003;142(3):253-8.

[21] Wood RJ, Volek JS, Liu Y, Shachter NS, Contois JH, Fernandez ML. Carbohydrate restriction alters lipoprotein metabolism by modifying VLDL, LDL, and HDL subfraction distribution and size in overweight men. J Nutr. 2006;136(2):384-389.

[22] Nordmann AJ, Nordmann A, Briel M, Keller B, Yancy WS Jr, Brehm, BJ, Bucher HC. Effects of low-carbohydrate vs low-fat diets on weight loss and cardiovascular risk factors. A meta-analysis of randomized controlled trials. Arch Intern Med. 2006;166(3):285-93.

[23] Bueno NB, de Melo IS, de Oliveira SL, da Rocha Ataide T. Very-low-carbohydrate ketogenic diet v. low-fat diet for long-term weight loss: a meta-analysis of randomized controlled trials. Br J Nutr. 2013;110(7):1178-87.

[24] Murphy P, Likhodii S, Nylen K, Burnham WM. The antidepressant properties of the ketogenic diet. Biol Physchiatry. 2004;56(12):981-3.

[25] El-Mallakh RS, Paskitti ME. The ketogenic diet may have mood-stabilizing properties. Med Hypotheses. 2001;57(6):724-726.

[26] D'Anci KE, Watts KL, Kanarek RB, Taylor HA. Low-carbohydrate weight-loss diets. Effects on cognition and mood. Appetite. 2009;52(1):96-103.

[27] Westman EC, Yancy WS Jr, Mavropoulos JC, Marquart M, McDuffie JR. The effect of a low-carbohydrate, ketogenic diet versus a low-glycemic index diet on glycemic control in type 2 diabetes mellitus. Nutr Metab (Lond). 2008;5:36.

[28] Feinman RD, Pogozelski WK, Astrup A, et al. Dietary carbohydrate restriction as the first approach in diabetes management: critical review and evidence base [published correction appears in Nutrition. 2019 Jun;62:213]. Nutrition. 2015;31(1):1-13.

29 Boden G, Sargrad K, Homko C, Mozzoli M, Stein TP. Effect of a low-carbohydrate diet on appetite, blood glucose levels, and insulin resistance in obese patients with type 2 diabetes. Ann Intern Med. 2005;142(6):403-411.

30 Yancy WS Jr, Foy M, Chalecki AM, Vernon MC, Westman EC. A low-carbohydrate, ketogenic diet to treat type 2 diabetes. Nutr Metab (Lond). 2005;2:34.

31 Hendricks EJ, Greenway FL, Westman EC, Gupta AK. Blood pressure and heart rate effects, weight loss and maintenance during long-term phentermine pharmacotherapy for obesity. Obesity (Silver Spring). 2011;19(12):2351-2360.

32 D'Andrea Meira I, Romão TT, Pires do Prado HJ, Krüger LT, Pires MEP, da Conceição PO. Ketogenic Diet and Epilepsy: What We Know So Far. Front Neurosci. 2019;13:5.

33 Murphy P. Use of the ketogenic diet as a treatment for epilepsy refractory to drug treatment. Expert Rev Neurother. 2005;5(6):769-775.

34 Zare M, Okhovat AA, Esmaillzadeh A, Mehvari J, Najafi MR, Saadatnia M. Modified Atkins diet in adult with refractory epilepsy: A controlled randomized clinical trial. Iran J Neurol. 2017;16(2):72-77.

35 Cheng B, Yang X, An L, Gao B, Liu X, Liu S. Ketogenic diet protects dopaminergic neurons against 6-OHDA neurotoxicity via up-regulating glutathione in a rat model of Parkinson's disease. Brain Res. 2009;1286:25-31.

36 Zhao Z, Lange DJ, Voustianiouk A, et al. A ketogenic diet as a potential novel therapeutic intervention in amyotrophic lateral sclerosis. BMC Neurosci. 2006;7:29.

37 McDonald TJW, Cervenka MC. Ketogenic Diets for Adult Neurological Disorders. Neurotherapeutics. 2018;15(4):1018-1031.

38 Verrotti A, Iapadre G, Pisano S, Coppola G. Ketogenic diet and childhood neurological disorders other than epilepsy: an overview. Expert Rev Neurother. 2017;17(5):461-473.

39 De Souza, R. J. et al. (2015) Intake of saturated and trans unsaturated fatty acids and risk of all cause mortality, cardiovascular disease, and type 2 diabetes: systematic review and meta analysis of observational studies. BMJ 351:h3978.

[40] Blasbalg, T. L. et al. (2011) Changes in consumption of omega 3 and omega 6 fatty acids in the United States during the 20th century. Am. J. Clin. Nutr. 93, 950 – 962.

[41] Kresser (2004) The Paleo Cure.

[42] Becerra-Tomas N, Diaz-Lopez A, Rosique-Esteban N, et al. Legume consumption is inversely associated with type 2 diabetes incidence in adults: a prospective assessment from the PREDIMED study. Clinical Nutrition. Mar 2017;S0261-5614(17)30106-1.

[43] Fowler SPG, Williams K, Hazuda HP. Diet soda intake is associated with long-term increases in waist circumference in a bi-ethnic cohort of older adults: The San Antonio Longitudinal Study of Aging. J Am Geriatr Soc. 2015;63(4):708–715.

[44] Weston M, Taylor KL, Batterham AM, Hopkins WG. Effects of low-volume high-intensity interval training (HIT) on fitness in adults: A meta-analysis of controlled and non-controlled trials. Sports Med. 2014;44(7):1005-17.

[45] Schleppenbach LN, Ezer AB, Gronemus SA, et al. Speed- and circuit-based high-intensity interval training on recovery oxygen consumption. Int J Exerc Sci. 2017;10(7):942-3.

[46] Puig-Ribera A, Bort-Roig J, Gine-Gerriga M, et al. Impact of a workplace 'sit less, move more' program on efficiency-related outcomes of office employees. BMC Public Health. May 2017;17(1):455.

[47] Coulson JC, McKenna J, Field M. Exercising at work and self-reported work performance. International Journal of Workplace Health Management. 2008;1(3):176-97.

[48] Hogan CL, Mata J, Carstensen LL. Exercise holds immediate benefits for affect and cognition in younger and older adults. Psychol Aging. Jun 2013;28(2):587-94.

[49] Mata J, Hogan CL, Joormann J. Acute exercise attenuates negative affect following repeated sad mood inductions in persons who have recovered from depression. J Abnorm Psychol. Feb 2013;122(1):45-50.

[50] Cosman F, de Beur SJ, LeBoff MS, et al. Clinician's guide to prevention and treatment of osteoporosis. Osteoporosis International. 2014;25:2359-81.

51 De Laet C, Kanis JA, Oden A, Johanson H, et al. Body mass index as a predictor of fracture risk: a meta-analysis. Osteoporos Int. 2005;16:1330-8.

52 Bagi CM, Edwards K, Berryman E. Metabolic syndrome and bone: pharmacologically induced diabetes has deleterious effect on bone in growing obese rats. Calcif Tissue Int. 2017 Dec 1.

53 Wong SK, Chin KY, Suhaimi FH, Ahmad F, et al. Osteoporosis is associated with metabolic syndrome induced by high-carbohydrate high-fat diet in a rat model. Biomed Phamacother. 2018 Feb;98:191-200.

54 Pirih F, Lu J, Bezouglaia O, Atti E, et al. Adverse effects of hyperlipidemia on bone regeneration and strength. J Bone Miner Res. 2012;27:309-18.

55 Bastos MF, Brilhante FV, Bezerra JP, Silva CA, et al. Trabecular bone area and bone healing in spontaneously hypertensive rats: a histometric study. Braz Oral Res. 2010;24:170-6.

56 Liu W, Zhu X, Wang Q, Wang L. Hyperglycemia induces endoplasmic reticulum stress-dependent CHOP expression in osteoblasts. Exp Ther Med. 2013;5:1289-92.

57 Halade GV, Rahman MM, Williams PJ, Fernandes G. High fat diet-induced animal model of age-associated obesity and osteoporosis. J Nutr Biochem. 2010;21:1162-9.

58 Kim JH, Choi HJ, Kim MJ, Shin CS, et al. Fat mass is negatively associated with bone mineral content in Koreans. Osteoporos Int. 2012;23(7):2009-16.

59 Zhou J, Zhang Q, Yuan X, Wang J, et al. Association between metabolic syndrome and osteoporosis: a meta-analysis. Bone. 2013;57(1):30-5.

60 Kim T, Park S, Pak YS, Lee S, et al. Association between metabolic syndrome and bone mineral density in Korea: the fourth Korea national health and nutrition examination survey (KNHANES IV), 2008. J Bone Miner Metab. 2013;31(6)652-62.

61 Muka T, Trajanoska K, Kiefte-de Jong JC, Oei L, et al. The association between metabolic syndrome, bone mineral density, hip bone geometry and fracture risk: the Rotterdam study. PLoS One. 2016;10(6):e0129116.

62 Eckstein N, Buchmann N, Demuth I, Steinhagen-Thiessen E, et al. Association between metabolic syndrome and bone mineral density-

data from the Berlin aging study II (BASE-II). Gerentology. 2016;62(3):337-44.

[63] Kim H, Oh HJ, Choi H, Choi WH, et al. The association between bone mineral density and metabolic syndrome: a Korean population-based study. J Bone Miner Metab. 2013;31(5):571-8.

[64] Oldroyd A, Mitchell K, Bukhari M. The prevalence of osteoporosis in an older population with very high body mass index: evidence for an association. Int J Clin Pract. 2014;68(6):771-4.

[65] El Maghraoui A, Rezqi A, El Mrahi S, Sadni S, et al. Osteoporosis, vertebral fractures and metabolic syndrome in postemenopausal women. BMC Endocr Disord. 2014;14:93

[66] Sozen T, Basaran NC, Tinazil M, Ozisi L. Musculoskeletal problems in diabetes mellitus. Eur J Rheumatol. 2018;5(4);258-65.

ABOUT THE AUTHORS

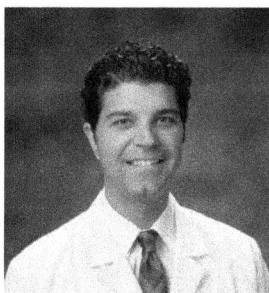

DR. JOHN RIEHL attended medical school in Philadelphia, PA, at Temple University School of Medicine where he obtained a robust clinical experience and foundation in medicine. He then performed his orthopedic surgery residency in central Pennsylvania at Geisinger Medical Center. It was here that Dr. Riehl and Dr. Lutton first met, and a dynamic partnership was formed. Dr. Lutton and Dr. Riehl discovered very early on their propensity to work well together and accomplish difficult tasks, from complex surgeries to writing and publishing. After residency Dr. Riehl completed subspecialty training in complex trauma/fracture care at Orlando Regional Medical Center. After his training was completed, Dr. Riehl went into practice at the University of Louisville where he was an assistant professor of orthopedic surgery and was quickly made the associate residency program director as a result of his affinity for teaching medical students, residents, and fellows. Dr. Riehl received the award of the Best Faculty Educator of the residents two years in a row while at the University of Louisville. He then took his orthopedic skills to Florida and the gulf coast for nearly seven years. During that time, he also began working at a trauma center in eastern Kentucky as the director of orthopedic trauma.

Dr. Riehl currently lives and practices in Dallas/Fort Worth, TX. He has been part of clinical faculty at universities throughout his career where he has contributed to research and education. He works as an editor/reviewer for three orthopedic journals and an industry leading orthopedic educational website. Dr. Riehl has developed and implemented treatment protocols at several institutions throughout his career that have improved patient care. He now brings his training and education, along with the expertise of Dr. Lutton, to you to help you on your path to better health.

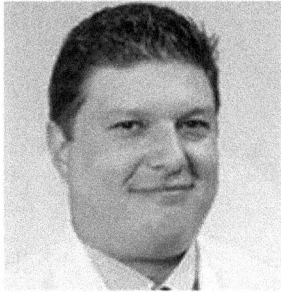

DR. JEFFREY LUTTON was born and raised in Pottstown, PA. He attended college at Villanova University where he majored in Chemistry and was awarded the prestigious Mendel Medallion. Dr. Lutton played rugby while at college and was very active in volunteer endeavors. He attended medical school at Georgetown University with the plans of becoming a cardiologist, but fell in love with orthopedic surgery in his third year of medical school and those plans changed significantly. Dr. Lutton was introduced to the concept of *cura personalis* (Latin for *care of the whole person*) while at Georgetown and that has formed the foundation of his medical practice to this day. He underwent specialty training in orthopedic surgery at Geisinger Medical Center where he encountered many great mentors who pushed him to reach his potential and helped him to establish strong surgical skills. At Geisinger he was challenged to always strive for evidence-based practice and to stay on the cutting edge of orthopedic surgery.

Dr. Lutton went into practice in 2011 in Chambersburg, PA and quickly became a local sensation. He has touched the lives and helped many members of his community. Recently he accepted a position at The Guthrie Clinic in the Southern Tier of New York where he will be helping to start a new orthopedic surgery residency program. Dr. Lutton (as is the case with Dr. Riehl) is known by many of his patients and colleagues to have a superb bedside manner. He is highly skilled in joint replacement surgery and general musculoskeletal care. Dr. Lutton and Dr. Riehl genuinely care about people and their general health, which has inspired them to bring the Intelligent Carb lifestyle to you.

www.ingramcontent.com/pod-product-compliance
Lightning Source LLC
Chambersburg PA
CBHW052044270326
41931CB00012B/2618